The M

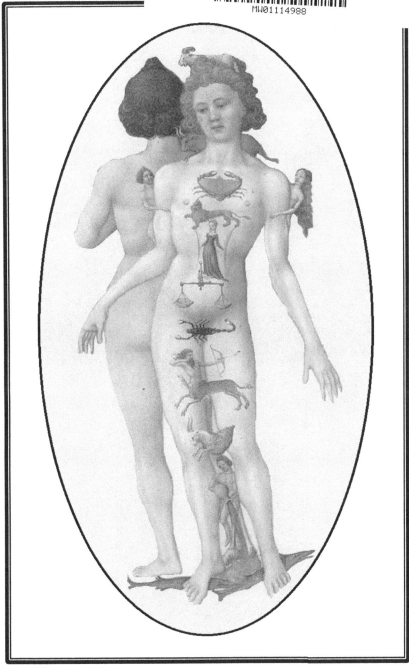

The Metaphysical Diet

By

B R Taylor

2018

Preface

The idea for this book came about from my concern towards the growing number of people suffering from obesity and severe weight problems. I had a suspicion that most people's habitual behaviour towards eating three meals a day was contributing to their dilemma. My knowledge of astrology together with universal wisdom and cosmic cycles convinced me that if we go back to some of humanities traditional ways of eating then a possible solution may be found. After months of research concerning this topic a solution was found, it is now known as '*The Metaphysical Diet*'.

Contents

The Metaphysical Diet

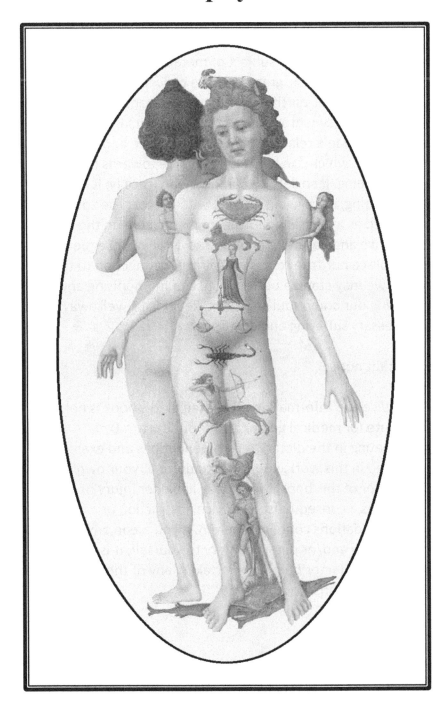

Introduction

Astrology is the *"Language of the Gods"*, and to understand its profound poetical secrets will help promote deeper awareness towards the subject of metaphysics (beyond the physical). With a basic grasp of these concepts one's physical experience on this earthly plane can be enhanced. The zodiac contains many synchronised secrets to universal wisdom concerning man's relationship towards nature and the macrocosm, which can be used as a guide towards harmony and well being. If society is to improve holistically, it must go back to being, once again, in tune with nature. The zodiac can be viewed as a diagrammatic benchmark between the human experience and nature's rhythms and cycles. Consequently, if we embrace our true roots and spiritual connection to these cycles, we may stand a better chance of harmonising and balancing our body, soul and spirit, keeping us well away from unnecessary suffering and dis-ease.

Important notice:

The advice and information presented in this book is no substitute for medical guidance by your doctor. By participating in the dietary recommendations and exercises contained in this work, you agree to do so at your own risk. The author of this book is in no way liable for injury or illness suffered as a consequence of advice, instruction or recommendations contained herein. If you are in any doubt as to the safety and/or possible injury to yourself, it is advised to consult your doctor before undertaking any of the recommendations.

Chapter 1. The importance of astrology

Astrology/applied astronomy is the oldest surviving language still in use today. Its glyphs, signs and form remain relatively unchanged from the days of ancient Sumer and dynastic Egypt. The Sumerians recorded their knowledge of the planets and constellations on clay tablets which date back over 5000 years. Their astrological system influenced the rest of the civilised world, making its way into Egypt, Rome and throughout the modern world we inhabit today.[1]

The reason why astrology is so important is because it identifies and maps cosmic cycles giving meaning and understanding to the human conscious relationship between the macrocosm, the microcosm and the Logos, basically identifying our true relationship with nature. Ancient myths and legends tell us that astronomy and astrology were given to humanity by the Titan God Atlas before the great deluge which destroyed Atlantis. It truly is the language of the Gods. The zodiac is presented in code form, where only a hand-full of readers have the experience and ability to decipher it accurately. Consequently, the further we deviate from its profound wisdom the greater chance we have of falling out of sync with nature's cycles, bringing forth dis-harmony and dis-ease upon our latest physical incarnation.

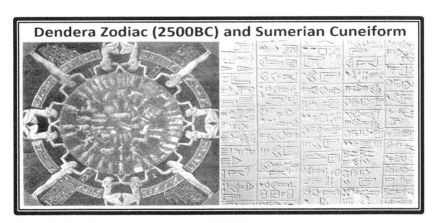
Dendera Zodiac (2500BC) and Sumerian Cuneiform

When we buy a new car, computer or kitchen appliance, these items usually come with a user manual, explaining how they work, and how to get the best out of them, in a safe and user friendly manner. Unfortunately, when a baby is born, no such information is offered, leaving most parents guessing about the child's strengths, weaknesses and personality type. However, if parents understood the value of an astrological birth chart, and how to read one, they could be one step closer towards understanding the child's natural and karmic relationship with the cosmos and the world he/she has just entered into. Simply put, the child's birth chart is a diagrammatic record of the position of the planets, in the heavens, at its moment of birth. This fixes planetary and cosmic energy, of various aspects and signs, within the child's biology and karmic disposition, giving the infant a unique personality of its own. Once this is understood, the child's strengths and weaknesses can be progressively assessed as it develops and interacts with future transiting planetary cycles within its new physical environment.

From an astrological perspective each planet in our solar system has its own individual character trait. The planets were thought to be the Gods of the ancient world, a world of polytheistic star and planet worship, considered by some, to be the Elohim.

In Genesis 1:1, it refers to the Elohim creating the heavens and the Earth. The word Elohim is a Hebrew plural term meaning more than one god.

In the beginning Elohim created heaven and earth. - Genesis 1:1 (NOG)

"Elohim is a grammatically plural noun for "gods" or "deity" in Biblical Hebrew." - Wikipedia "Elohim"

This is also backed up by Genesis 1:26, in which "us" and "our" are used, referring to more than one god.

Then God said, "Let us make mankind in our image, in our likeness." - Genesis 1:26 (NIV)

We live in an electric universe where the electromagnetic effects of the Elohim on our physical biology are tangible aspects of nature's cycles. Consequently, when the Sun appears on the horizon it marks the start of a new day and the beginning of a new zodiac cycle. In ancient Egypt the Sun's electromagnetic energetic influence on human biology was referred to as Horus. So at 6am Horus was seen rising up lighting the sky on the Horizon (Horus-rising). The Egyptians understood the profound influence the Sun's position had on our physical behaviour. It has always been regarded as the energy source behind our focal consciousness, promoting and energising us to awaken from the world of sleep, a world within the spiritual subconscious, and as it slowly appears in the morning it spreads its rays, illuminating all that lay in its path.

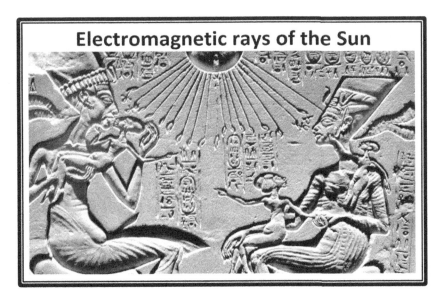
Electromagnetic rays of the Sun

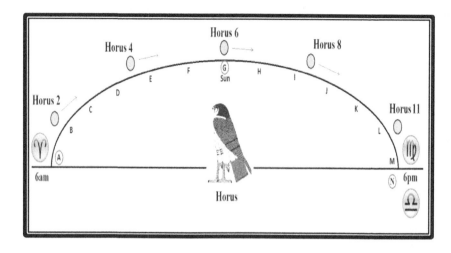

As civilisation evolved, moving from the Age of Aries into the Piscean Age, Christianity re-branded the ancient concept of Horus's angle in the sky, personifying it as Archangel Michael. It is really the angle of the planet or luminary in the sky, the ang of El.

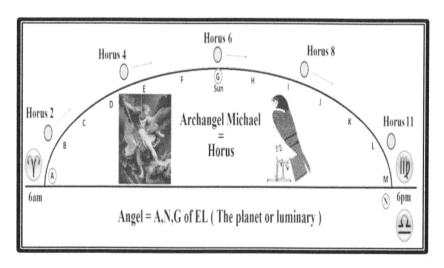

Consequently, each Archangel represents a different planet as it moves across the heavens. It is therefore understandable, in this electric universe, to find all the Archangel's names ending with 'el'.

Sun = Archangel Michael
Moon = Archangel Gabriel
Mars = Archangel Samael
Mercury = Archangel Raphael
Jupiter = Archangel Sachiel
Venus = Archangel Haniel
Saturn = Archangel Cassiel

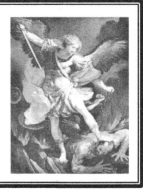

With this knowledge, it is possible to identify the Sun's energetic influence on human biology during the course of the day, as it progresses across the sky. But first a basic overall understanding of astrological signs, glyphs and planets is needed to put it all in perspective.

Sun	Self, Will, Focal Consciousness	I Will Act	⊙
Moon	Emotion, Needs, Feelings, Subconscious	I React	☾
Mercury	Communication, Mind	I Communicate	☿
Venus	Love, Liking, Pleasure	I Harmonise	♀
Mars	Physical energy, Action	I Assert	♂
Jupiter	Expansion, Abundance	I Expand	♃
Saturn	Time, Seriousness, Discipline, Restriction	I Control	♄
Uranus	Revolution, Change	I Deviate	⛢
Neptune	Dreams, Illusions	I Refine	♆
Pluto	Transformation	I Transform	♇

When we analyse the individual astrological glyphs for the planets within our solar system we find they are essentially made up of various combinations from three basic components, the soul, the spirit and the physical.

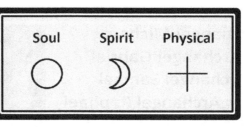

Soul	Spirit	Physical

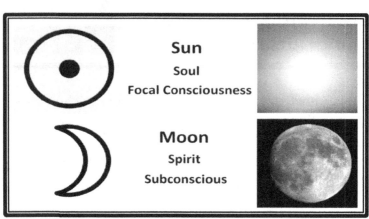

Sun
Soul
Focal Consciousness

Moon
Spirit
Subconscious

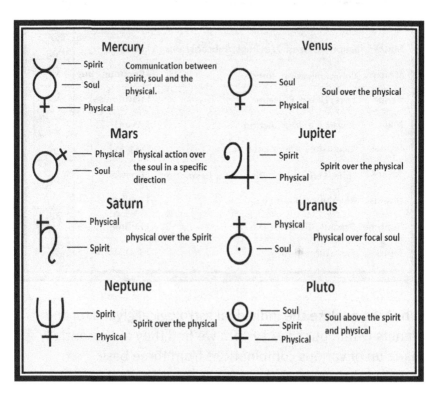

Mercury
— Spirit
— Soul
— Physical
Communication between spirit, soul and the physical.

Venus
— Soul
— Physical
Soul over the physical

Mars
— Physical
— Soul
Physical action over the soul in a specific direction

Jupiter
— Spirit
— Physical
Spirit over the physical

Saturn
— Physical
— Spirit
physical over the Spirit

Uranus
— Physical
— Soul
Physical over focal soul

Neptune
— Spirit
— Physical
Spirit over the physical

Pluto
— Soul
— Spirit
— Physical
Soul above the spirit and physical

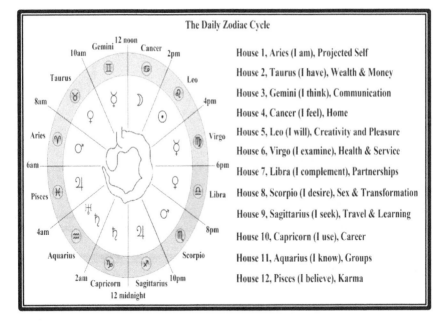

The Daily Zodiac Cycle

House 1, Aries (I am), Projected Self

House 2, Taurus (I have), Wealth & Money

House 3, Gemini (I think), Communication

House 4, Cancer (I feel), Home

House 5, Leo (I will), Creativity and Pleasure

House 6, Virgo (I examine), Health & Service

House 7, Libra (I complement), Partnerships

House 8, Scorpio (I desire), Sex & Transformation

House 9, Sagittarius (I seek), Travel & Learning

House 10, Capricorn (I use), Career

House 11, Aquarius (I know), Groups

House 12, Pisces (I believe), Karma

It is also important, at this stage, to have a basic grasp of the difference between the focal conscious mind/soul and the subconscious mind/spirit, along with knowledge of how that consciousness interacts with the macrocosm and universal consciousness/Logos. Our ancestors believed in a triad of consciousness underpinning the human experience, with the focal mind being only a fraction of the capacity and scope of the subconscious. Modern science supports this impressive potential within the subconscious, suggesting it is anywhere between 70-95% of the mind's overall capacity.[2] Simply put, the small focal conscious mind can be defined as what we are focusing our attention on at any given moment. Whereas, the subconscious is the internal emotional part of our mind, the background store deep within us, remembering everything we ever experienced like a digital hard drive inside a computer. While the focal mind is restricted, by physical constraints of time and space, the subconscious connects to the spirit realm giving it almost unlimited potential and scope outside material constraints.

8

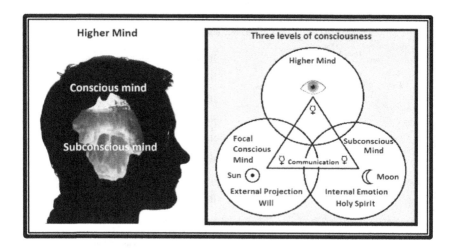

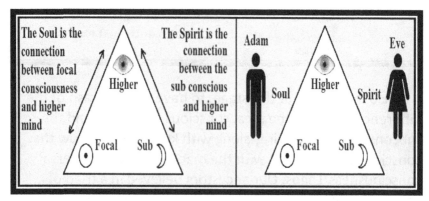

If we look at the zodiac chart as a single daily cycle, from the perspective of common human activities, starting the day at 6am in Aries, we see some interesting correlations between the zodiac and human behaviour.

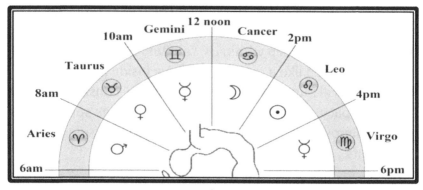

6am – 8am, Aries the ram, ruled by Mars. The start of a new day. As the Sun appears on the horizon, most people awaken and come back into focal consciousness, they lift their heads off the pillow and once again become aware of themselves, from the head down. Many males experience a peak in testosterone, giving rise to an early morning erection, known as a morning glory.[3] When one analyses the glyph for Mars, we see a circle with what looks like, an erection, the circle represents the focal consciousness, the soul and the masculine. Many people leave the house and head for work during this time, frantically fighting their way through the morning traffic like competing rams or sheeple.

8am – 10am, Taurus the bull, ruled by Venus. Most people settle into their daily routine at this time, like the bull of Taurus, they place themselves in their chosen field. They will use their voices to greet one another, converse and arrange their daily agenda.

10am – 12noon, Gemini the twins, ruled by Mercury, the planet of communication. 11am is the most common time, in the US, for meetings to take place.[4] Being the sign associated with the arms and hands we see many people with practical skills putting their arms and hands to work, in an overall productive 2 hours before lunch.

12noon – 2pm, Cancer the crab, ruled by the Moon. The Moon is internal sensitivity, seeking emotional fulfilment. The Moon rules various areas of the body, including the chest, the breast, the stomach and the alimentary canal. Here we see most people taking their lunch break, satisfying their inner feelings of hunger, they also take time out to internalise.

2pm – 4pm, Leo the lion, ruled by the Sun. In many countries, with the Sun at its hottest, people take a siesta. Many traditional cultures would go home at this time and sleep for a few hours. There is an old saying "to sleep like a lion", this is because lions can sleep up to 20 hours a day if necessary.[5] Various studies have been carried out which suggest the best time to take an afternoon nap is between 2-3pm.[6]

4pm – 6pm, Virgo the virgin, ruled by Mercury. This is the house of health and service to others. Studies have shown that this is the best time for exercise, due to the overall body temperature increasing throughout the day, along with heart rate and blood pressure falling, this makes late afternoon the best time for physical exercise.[7]

6pm – 8pm, Libra the balancing scales, ruled by Venus, the house of partnerships and marriage. During this time the Sun fades, disappearing over the horizon, most people's working day has come to an end, and many of them make their way home to be with their partners or loved ones.

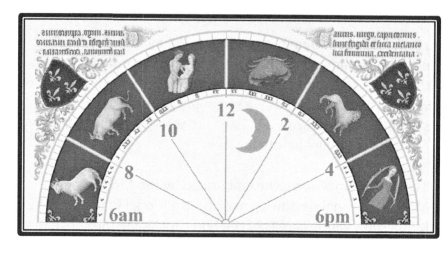

From this we can see how the zodiac, reflecting harmonious natural cycles, would suggest that the best time for eating should be between 12 noon and 2pm. This is because the ruling planet of Cancer is the Moon, the planet associated with internal emotions, needs and sensitivity. It represents the subconscious, our habitual nature along with the stomach.

Consequently, the zodiac is giving us the perfect window of opportunity to break our morning fast by eating something nutritious each day.

The Moon and the Subconscious

The Moon, has for thousands of years, been connected to, and represented by water, the feminine, the spirit realm, darkness and the subconscious. Consequently, it is not surprising to find the same 70/30 ratio in other areas of nature concerning water and the subconscious.

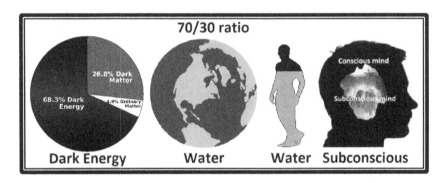

From an astrological perspective the Moon represents the following:

● Deepest personal needs.
● Habitual behaviour.
● Reactions and instincts.
● Subconscious mind.
● Feelings, emotions and intuition.
● Spirit.
● Inner child.
● Responsive, receptive and reflective.

While the Sun represents our wants in the physical world of the focal consciousness, the Moon reflects our needs. There is an old profound saying within the ancient world of esoteric wisdom. It tells us that the universe gives us what we need, not necessarily what we want. This is because the subconscious, connected to the spirit realm and universal consciousness knows us better than we know ourselves, and many of our wants in this physical world of the focal consciousness are the result of subtle suggestions socially engineered for, and by, corporate motives, clouding our judgment between wants and needs.

With all this in mind, it seems plausible, at this point, to speculate on the possibility of a profound link between the Moon, the subconscious and our habitual eating habits. A link which if understood and properly utilised, could promote discipline over one's habitual needs concerning those eating habits.

The focal consciousness of humanity shares a common collective within the physical realm of human behaviour, our souls interact on a biological level, from the soles of our feet to the top of our heads, within the limitations of spatial awareness. Our subconscious, the dominant part of our mind also interacts within a collective, outside the constraints of time and space, within the profound unlimited scope of the spirit realm. This huge capacity of consciousness interacting on a subconscious level is the engine of our perception of reality. The subconscious being 70% of our minds capacity, and also part of a collective, is responsible for the potential offerings of energetic frequencies surrounding our physical reality. From that external potential our focal consciousness homes in on matching frequencies which harmonise with its specific disposition at any given time. This is how the feedback loop is created and how we perceive reality. Whoever controls our subconscious controls the game, they dictate the boundaries within the potential to our perceived reality through limiting and controlling the scope of the subconscious.

When a child is born, for the first two years of its life, the child's conscious mind is in, what is referred to as, the delta state, this is deep sleep or coma like consciousness. Between two and six the child's brain activity increases into the theta state, this is very much like being in a hypnotic trance, where the subconscious is fully open and acts like a sponge, downloading massive amounts of unfiltered information, perceptions and experiences about the world and how it works, mixing the real world with the child's imagination. This is when we are programmed, during those early years, with our own unique beliefs, a reflection of our immediate surroundings, our parents behaviour, and our interaction with the community. We are essentially programmed before our focal conscious mind has developed to a point at which it can filter new information entering the subconscious. Consequently, most people spend the rest of their lives with beliefs and habitual behavioural patterns which they had no say in or had very little control over. For the first seven years of a child's life both hemispheres of the brain are working together.[8] As they develop, specific thought processes will eventually take place in specific hemispheres, giving rise to the mature mind of the adult.

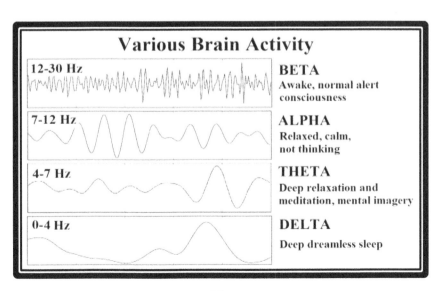

Various Brain Activity

12-30 Hz	**BETA** Awake, normal alert consciousness
7-12 Hz	**ALPHA** Relaxed, calm, not thinking
4-7 Hz	**THETA** Deep relaxation and meditation, mental imagery
0-4 Hz	**DELTA** Deep dreamless sleep

The subconscious can be compared to a computer's internal workings. At birth you come into this world with a specific karmic disposition, influenced by the orientation of universal and planetary energies. This could be viewed as the computers Central Processing Unit, whereas all a person's habitual beliefs would be the software, downloaded in the first seven years of life. The software can be reprogrammed but the CPU is there to stay. This can go some way towards explaining why some people have easier lives than others. Each of us starts off with unique CPU karmic mapping, added to this is the software downloaded during those formative years, from then on you are on your own, master over your perception of the world, while the planetary transits continue to influence the CPU, it is up to the individual to make updates to that initial software.

The problem most people experience, as they develop, is that their focal conscious thought processes, of wants, needs and desires, don't always run in harmony with the subconscious mind's habitual beliefs, they sometimes coexist in conflict. Because the subconscious is responsible for 70% of the mind and most of our perceived reality, the focal mind's wishes, in the physical world, are not always fulfilled. It takes a great deal of effort for the small focal mind, to manifest your desires in the physical realm, especially if it is running contrary to the massive capacity of the subconscious.

The focal conscious mind acts as a spotlight on an unlimited array of possibilities offered by the collective subconscious. Our individual subconscious is our karmic disposition together with our programmed beliefs, and because the focal conscious minds capacity is so small compared to the subconscious, anyone wishing to influence their perception of reality, should really start by targeting the subconscious for change, as opposed to battling through their inharmonious gremlins in the physical realm, relying solely on the focal conscious mind.

Most people's minds are full of chatter, the monkey mind is a constant stream of random thoughts, images and reflections of events and scenarios. Many of these thoughts are self-sabotaging, negative rhetoric, reinforcing Saturnian pessimism, frustrations and restrictions. This must be dealt with early and neutralised, before it grows into a reoccurring problem, having the potential to attach itself to the subconscious as a new negative habitual belief system.

Through the process of regular meditation, one learns to quieten the mind, turning away from monkey mind chatter towards stillness. One major benefit of meditation is its ability to allow reprogramming of the subconscious with new positive beliefs, which run in harmony with the focal minds dreams, wishes and desires. Everything in this world is possible, not just for a few, but for all. The only thing holding most of us back is our inner habitual beliefs running in conflict with our physical aspirations; yet most people in the western world have no idea how to rectify this problem, which could lead towards a better life of fulfilment, happiness, success and well-being.

To live one's life by solely relying upon the focal conscious mind, in the physical realm, to guide and solve all life's problems, while ignoring the vast capacity of the subconscious; is like having one hundred radio stations, but only ever tuning into a handful. When the focal and subconscious are finally working in harmony, your life's potential is limitless, even to the point of illumination.

A good analogy to use, when trying to understand this whole concept, is to visualise a man riding on the back of a large elephant. The man represents the focal mind, and the elephant is the subconscious. During the man's childhood, the elephant is told to go on a journey, through the forest, from A to B. This does not cause a problem during the early years of the man's life, but as he grows up and starts to think for himself, he finds his new wants, needs and desires are not in tune with the elephant, he now wants to go from A to Z. But the little man, only a fraction of the strength and size of the elephant, finds it difficult to persuade the elephant to go in this new direction; and in order to create a new path he has to fight, all alone, with the elephant and the forest simultaneously. One night the man has a dream where he is shown how to speak a new language allowing him to talk to the elephant; over the next few days the man and the elephant begin to communicate and start working together in harmony. He convinces the elephant to change course, to the new destination of A to Z. From then on the man no longer had to struggle with the forest or the elephant, he let the enormous and powerful animal do all the hard work while he sat on its back and enjoyed the ride.

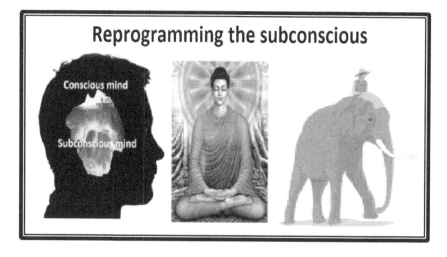

The elephant analogy used to describe the subconscious is an interesting one, because in the Hindu tradition the elephant headed God Ganesha has many similar characteristics to the human subconscious mind.

● Invokes order to remove obstacles.

- His large pot belly is said to contain the universe, past, present and future.
- He has paranormal powers.
- A snake girdles around his pot belly (snakes are nocturnal hunters, and are used to represent the subconscious).
- He has childlike innocence and behaviour, just like the subconscious, which was fully open when we were children. Consequently, when we communicate with the subconscious we have to talk to it as though it was a 6 year old child, in the present tense.
- He also represents the divine consciousness.
- The rope Ganesha holds in his left (subconscious) hand, is the weapon used to remove obstacles.
- He rides on top of a mouse or rat, which represents the human focal conscious mind.
- He symbolises life cycles which challenge us to expand our consciousness.

Once you have Ganesha, or your subconscious elephant, on the same side as your focal conscious mind's dreams, wishes and desires, anything becomes possible.

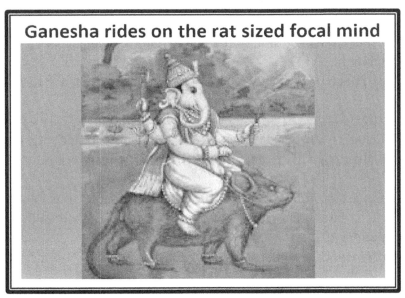

Ganesha rides on the rat sized focal mind

Notes for chapter 1

(1) Demetra George, Sumerian astrology, historical astrology, 2018.
http://www.historicalastrology.com/astrology-of-ancient-sumer/

(2) Marianne Szegedy-Maszak, Mysteries of the mind, Your unconscious is making your everyday decisions.
http://www.auburn.edu/~mitrege/ENGL2210/USNWR-mind.htm
l

(3) Nocturnal Penile Tumescence, Wikipedia,
https://en.wikipedia.org/wiki/Nocturnal_penile_tumescence

(4) Nicholas C. Romano, Jr. Jay F. Nunamaker, Jr.   Meeting Analysis: Findings from Research and Practice, Page 1, Proceedings of the 34th Hawaii International Conference on System Sciences – 2001.
http://citeseerx.ist.psu.edu/viewdoc/download?doi=10.1.1.570.6650&rep=rep1&type=pdf

(5) Sleep habits of lions, National Sleep Foundation,
https://sleep.org/articles/sleep-habits-of-lions/

(6) What's the best time of the day to nap? National Sleep Foundation,
https://sleep.org/articles/whats-the-best-time-of-the-day-to-nap
/

(7) Claudine Morgan, When`s the best time to workout? July 4th 2016, http://greatist.com/fitness/whats-best-time-work-out

(8) Bruce Lipton, 7 ways to reprogram your subconscious mind, How to create the honeymoon effect every day. Cheap health revolution. 2014,
http://www.cheap-health-revolution.com/honeymoon-effect.ht
ml

Chapter 2. The power of the subconscious

We have already established in chapter 1 how the subconscious is initially programmed during the early years of a person's life, a time of great sensitivity to environmental stimuli. Consequently, seeds planted within the subconscious during this time are either watered down or neglected depending upon future focus and attention. The elephant has essentially been given his coordinates and is now well on his way.

In a capitalist system based around consumerism, the desire for perpetual growth is a major consideration when socially engineering the minds of the next generation into being needy towards your products and services. If seeds desiring corporate products can be sown within the child's subconscious at a very young age, the prospect of recruiting a future consumer towards a corporations products is greatly increased.

A large part of advertising for corporate consumerism is designed and targeted at the minds of children, at an early age, with Christmas and Thanks Giving being major events which teach children to associate joy, happiness, worth and affection with bright coloured toys, sweets, sodas and overindulgence. The more of the five senses stimulated during this process the deeper the seeds become grounded within the garden of the subconscious, leading to some deep rooted habitual behavioral patterns. Once inside the subconscious those wants associated with the focal conscious mind become habitual needs within the subconscious. As the child develops and becomes a young adult, their wants and desires sometimes develop running contrary to early programming needs within the subconscious. People's habits usually take on similar formats to that of their parents and/or the environment which they find themselves brought up in. So how does someone go about changing unhealthy eating habits, which have been with them most of their lives?

Habits become destiny.

To have better control over one's life, these habits must be either encouraged or discouraged before they can influence a person's character and consequently their destiny. Using the zodiac to illustrate this, we can see how the thought, in the head, leads to the word in the throat, which promotes the act, leading to habit, character and destiny. Once the seed in the mind of the subconscious germinates, it becomes very difficult to remove it.

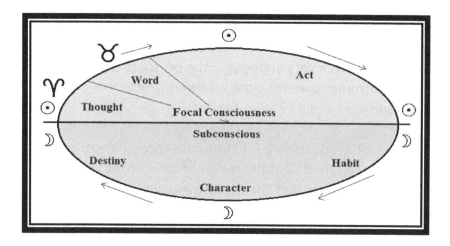

Reprogramming the subconscious

Considering the majority of one's subconscious programming took place before the age of 7, which set the stage for the individual's future eating habits, in order to reprogram it, one needs to recreate the same conditions which initially opened the door to the subconscious during those formative years.

"Give me a child until he is seven and I will show you the man." - Aristotle

Apart from hypnosis, meditation is one of the best ways to place the mind in the theta state, it is also important to recreate balance in thought between hemispheres, as with the mind of the child; this is known as hemi-sync. One way to achieve this is to cross one's legs and arms, as the left side of the brain controls the right side of the body and vice versa, this stimulates both hemispheres. Once this is achieved and the mind has become centred, repetition and positive affirmations can be offered as mantras in order to influence and reprogram the subconscious with new beliefs running in parallel to one's new goals. Because the subconscious is extremely powerful and is our spiritual connection to the higher mind collective; unlike the sequential focal mind, the subconscious has the ability to operate outside the constraints of time and space. With a new belief system in place, your perception of reality will change from within. People and events will seem coincidental, as the world around you seems to order itself towards your new objectives, illuminating those similar energies easily for the focal mind to home in on. This is how your dreams really do come true.

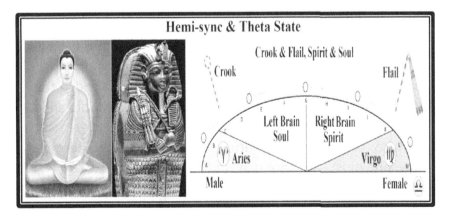

Positive affirmations and mantras

There are many ways to reprogram the subconscious, when trying to make changes as adults. Repetition is successful, but takes a while and many hours of dedication, it works by creating new automatic habits which are the domain of the subconscious. We learn our mathematical tables this way, reciting them off by heart without even having to think or engage the focal mind. To become the greatest version of yourself, in this limited lifetime, and to live a more fulfilled and happy life, one's internal programming must be in tune with those positive aspirations. If an individual desires a loving relationship, but has difficulty in manifesting this in their reality, it could be due to conflicting belief systems. A child may have, in its early years, harboured a belief of doubt and separation in the area of love, and may have difficulty not only trusting others, but also loving themselves. To rectify this a new belief must be downloaded into the subconscious, through repetition of positive mantras, one can stimulate the growth of a seed into a new belief system, while at the same time preventing any further nurturing of unwanted seeds. Once in the meditative state the person must convince the subconscious mind that he loves himself. He must repeat the mantra "I love myself", until it becomes a fixture in his habitual nature. It is very difficult to love others if one does not care much for one's self. Using this technique one can work on all areas of their lives until the subconscious is finally playing ball with the focal mind's latest aspirations. The mantra used must be simple, straight to the point and in the present tense, as though you are talking to a 6 year old child. It is no good reciting the words "I will be rich" because that is a future concept, and the future will never be in the here and now, one must say "I am rich" or " I am wealthy".

Positive Mantra		
I am happy	I love myself	I have lots of energy
I am wealthy	I love my life	I don't smoke
I am healthy	I love my career	I don't drink alcohol
I am slim	I love humanity	People like me

"Therefore I say unto you. What things soever ye desire, when ye pray, believe that ye receive them, and ye shall have them." - Mark 11:24 (KJV)

"Whatever your mind can conceive and believe the mind can achieve regardless of how many times you may have failed in the past." - Napoleon Hill

"As a single footstep will not make a path on the earth, so a single thought will not make a pathway in the mind. To make a deep physical path, we walk again and again. To make a deep mental path, we must think over and over the kind of thoughts we wish to dominate our lives." - Wilfred A Peterson

"Whether you think you can or think you can't, either way you are right." - Henry Ford

"Nurture your mind with great thoughts, for you will never go any higher than you think." - Benjamin Disraeli

"I attract to my life whatever I give my attention, energy and focus to, whether positive or negative." - Michael Losier

"The closer you come to knowing that you alone create the world of your experience, the more vital it becomes for you to discover just who is doing the creating." - Eric Micha'el Leventhal

"If you can believe that you can do it, the whole universe will conspire to help you." - Debasish Mridha

"If you change the way you look at things, the things you look at change." - Wayne Dyer

When trying to access the subconscious from our sequential focal conscious perspective, trapped by inherent boundaries of time and space, we come up against some difficulty. However, there are many ways to open this door, allowing us to reprogram the subconscious in order to plant new beliefs. The more of the five senses one can stimulate during the reprogramming phase, the greater the chance of success. Here are just a few ways to reprogram the subconscious mind:

- Positive affirmation: Repeating positive, present tense, statements, you can override negative thoughts and beliefs already lodged in the subconscious. Use simple positive phrases like "I am happy every day".
- Visualisation: Visualising your wants, needs and desires is a great way to stimulate the subconscious into accepting them as your new reality, conspiring with the universe to make it happen.
- Hypnosis: While extremely relaxed, with the mind in the theta state, the subconscious is open and easily reprogrammed from suggestions offered by a hypnotist.
- Subliminal audio/visual: The best time to use this method is when the mind is in the theta state, either at the start of the sleep cycle or towards the end.
- Meditation: This is one of the most popular ways to access the subconscious although it requires practice and dedication.
- Will power & habit: This is all part of repetition, with the will backing positive intent, through repetition, habits form, and from habits a new character is created.
- Auto-suggestion: Or self-suggestion is a simple way to influence the subconscious, new positive beliefs and intentions are repeatedly reinforced by the individual, until those old negative seeds and beliefs have withered away and perished.

Swimming is another great way to access and reprogram the subconscious; overlooked by many, this simple process does not get the attention it deserves. Considering water is synonymous with the spirit realm, the Moon and the subconscious, it seems a logical choice when choosing other forms of meditation and subconscious reprogramming. The action of swimming is a great opportunity to achieve moving meditation, while also stimulating many of the five senses, it really does tick all the right boxes.

- The swimming strokes are repetitive and rhythmic.
- The sensation of water flowing over the body, stimulates feelings.
- You hear the sound of the water in an isolated way.
- Helps to shut out external stimuli in a cocooning effect.
- While swimming you can focus your attention on your breathing.
- Activating hemi-sync by using both arms and legs to swim.
- Swimming can make you feel relaxed.

Once the swimmer has achieved a comfortable state of relaxation, with an easy, steady, repetitive stroke, positive mantra and visualisations can be introduced, this will open the door to the subconscious, allowing new seeds and beliefs to germinate.

Because the subconscious is a non-judgemental magnet to emotional stimuli, there is another practical way to influence it, a technique which has been known about for thousands of years. Being concerned with emotions, feelings, visualisation and sensory stimuli, there is no better way to energise all these right brain triggers than the emotionally charged orgasm. Many people make the time to create a self-induced orgasm, but are they wasting a valuable opportunity to influence their reality? Instead of focusing one's attention on factory made pornographic images, of all kinds of perversions, freely available on the internet; one could take the opportunity to use the orgasm as a mechanism to influence their physical wants, needs and desires, in a much boarder sense. So whatever one thinks about at the moment of orgasm, together with strong affirmative beliefs, one could sow some powerful seeds towards manifesting a whole new reality. This practice may need to come under the umbrella of repetition, in order to be certain of a positive outcome, and which could alter the meaning of the phrase "coming into money".[1]

This could also be the true meaning behind the ancient story of the genie in the magic lamp. When the lamp is rubbed the genie pops out and grants you a wish. Could the name genie be a derivative of genitals?

Meditation

Understanding the meaning of the word meditation is part of the puzzle, the etymology of the word suggests it came out of contemplation, devout preoccupation, devotions and prayer; from old French its roots were in thought, reflection and study; in Latin it is to think over, reflect and consider. It is also derived from the root "med", which is "to measure".

Meditation is constructed from "medi", and the Latin root for medi is "middle". Like all other words beginning with medi, they are concerned with the middle, words like:

- Medieval (Middle Ages).
- Mediocre (a task done in a mediocre way is average).
- Medium (the medium temperature is somewhere in the middle, a spiritual medium is a person who acts as a middle connection between the physical and the spiritual realms.

- Mediterranean (the middle sea), between Europe and Africa.
- Media (reporting from the middle of a story, who are supposed to be impartial, covering from the middle ground).
- Median (the middle number in a sequence of numbers).

Words ending with "ation" denotes an action or process.

- Notation (the act of structured written communication).
- Presentation (the act of presenting a new idea or topic to an audience).
- Illumination (the act of lighting up a source).

With this in mind we can assume that the art of meditation is a physical act in which a person is trying to reach some form of middle ground, concerning the mind and its thought processes. The mind is complicated and only partially understood. In our physical world of modern science, the combined metaphysical aspect of the human mind is overlooked in favour of tangible measurable units of focal consciousness. The world of the subconscious, which cannot be measured by physical instruments, is conveniently dismissed as a pseudoscience. Emotions cannot be measured; the love one has for one's parents or children has no mathematical scale or equation. However, this does not mean these emotions are fictitious, on the contrary, more people's lives are ruled by feelings of love and compassion than by Pythagoras's theorem or Einstein's theory of relativity.

Many modern forms of meditation, especially western meditation are the result of fads, fashions and commercial exploitation, brought about by a new wave of interest in ancient wisdom and philosophy. One must question everything, in order to find the right path for themselves. Each one of us is different, with unique karmic mapping, varying potentials of strengths and weaknesses. Consequently, any form of religion or culture with a one size fits all policy is not in the interest of the individual but for the benefit of the system of control growing up around them.

"Do not make meditation a complicated affair; it is really very simple and because it is simple it is very subtle. Its subtlety will escape the mind if the mind approaches it with all kinds of fanciful and romantic ideas. Meditation, really, is a penetration into the unknown, and so the known, the memory, the experience, the knowledge which it has acquired during the day, or during a thousand days, must end. For it is only a free mind that can penetrate into the very heart of the immeasurable. So meditation is both the penetration and the ending of the yesterday. The trouble begins when we ask how to end the yesterday. There is really no 'how.' The 'how' implies a method, a system and it is this very method and system that has conditioned the mind. Just see the truth of this. Freedom is necessary -not 'how' to be free. The 'how to be free' only enslaves you."- Jiddu Krishnamurti

"Meditation is one of the greatest arts in life, perhaps the greatest, and one cannot possibly learn it from anybody. That is the beauty of it. It has no technique and therefore no authority. When you learn about yourself, watch yourself, watch the way you walk, how you eat, what you say, the gossip, the hate, the jealousy, if you are aware of all that in yourself, without any choice, that is part of meditation. So meditation can take place when you are sitting in a bus or walking in the woods full of light and shadows, or listening to the singing of birds or looking at the face of your wife or child." - Jiddu krishnamurti

Buddhist monks or moonks are instantly recognisable in their orange robes and shaved heads. One explanation for their appearance can be deduced from their role as Moon watchers. Like all monks they are responsible for observing the cycles of the Moon. They shave their heads to symbolise the Moon and their orange robes represent the colour of the sky during sunset; a time when the Moon slowly becomes the dominant luminary in the sky. Unlike other religions the Buddhists don't focus on an artificially created holy day of the week, instead they base their holy days on the four main phases of the Moon: full moon, new moon and half-moons, harmonising their spiritual connection to nature. The moon days in the Theravadan calendar of Thailand are called "Wan Phra – (Monk Days)", all monks are expected to stay in the temple on these holy days.

Quotes from Buddha:

- The mind is everything. What you think you become.
- It is a man's own mind, not his enemy or foe, that lures him to evil ways.
- There is nothing so disobedient as an undisciplined mind, and there is nothing so obedient as a disciplined mind.
- Nothing can harm you as much as your own thoughts unguarded.
- Peace comes from within. Do not seek it without.
- There is no path to happiness: happiness is the path.

In Buddhism the word for meditation is "Bhavana", which means to "make grow" or "to develop". Meditation helps the individual develop a different awareness, along with the energy needed to transform unwanted mental habitual patterns, trapped within the subconscious. Buddha taught many different types of meditation, each targeting specific areas requiring attention, designed to overcome various issues and to develop specific psychological states of mind. The two most common forms are:

- Mindfulness of breath (anapana sati).
- Loving kindness meditation (metta bhavana).

By sitting quietly and focusing on the in-out movement of your breathing, you can train the mind to be in the space between thoughts, during which intruding thoughts will come and go, distracting you. By going back to focusing on your breathing, those unwanted thoughts should weaken and pass. With practice your ability to concentrate will improve, giving you moments of deep mental calm where inner peace will grow. Once the mindfulness of breath technique has been mastered, loving kindness meditation can be introduced. This form of meditation can influence the subconscious with positive words and affirmations, phrases like:

- I am wealthy, happy and healthy.
- I am peaceful and calm.
- I am protected from danger, anger and hatred.

Along with these positive affirmations, a good technique is to think of three people, one who you love, one who is neutral, and one who you have problems with, even dislike. In turn wish them all well, as you view them in your mind.

If this is done on a regular basis, the garden within the subconscious will begin to change, those old unwanted seeds of negative emotions like; hatred, bitterness, blame and resentment, will go un-watered, overshadowed by new seeds of positive emotions and affirmations, enabling a whole new habitual nature to grow from within.

It is my view that the whole concept of meditation is to bring one's mind and thoughts back into balance, towards the middle ground and away from extremes. If we look at the zodiac's houses, as a map of life's variety, and expressions of possibility; a balanced, measured mind should be somewhere in the centre, not around the edge at an extreme point. The further away from the middle, the further the mind is away from harmony and balance, preoccupied by one specific house's characteristics. The closer your thoughts are to the middle, the more balanced the mind becomes, and the more chance of peace in the space between thoughts. The saying "to be centred" is used much in modern society, to describe someone who is mentally balanced, even without a comprehensive metaphysical understanding of what it really means.

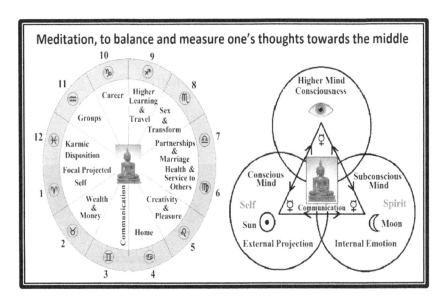

Meditation, to balance and measure one's thoughts towards the middle

It is also a process of balancing the focal conscious mind with the subconscious, in order to bring them in line with one another and away from conflict and disharmony. When both the focal and the subconscious are working together, the ability to influence one's own reality is greatly increased. With your thoughts you truly do make the world. This is all part of the enlightening process.

The posture for meditation is important in a number of ways. The legs are crossed to create a stable base for the spinal column to be naturally straight, one must feel comfortable in a relaxed unrestrained manner. The most popular positions are the full lotus, half lotus and the Burmese posture. The root chakra is placed firmly on the Earth, with the crown chakra positioned at the highest point. When one looks at the silhouette of the meditation position, it resembles a triangle, the three areas of consciousness. When one prays, they also create the triangle, by placing both hands together, pointing upwards. The joining of the hands is a physical expression of intention, joining or balancing both the left and right hemispheres, the focal and subconscious, in order to influence and manifest a new reality.

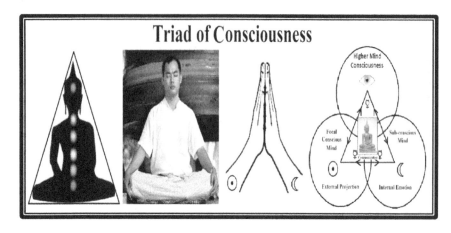

Collective meditation and prayer

"For where two or three are gathered together in my name, there am I in the midst of them." - Matthew 18:20

"You are helping us by praying for us. Then many people will give thanks because God has graciously answered so many prayers for our safety" - 2 Corinthians 1:11

Meditation and prayer work together as a mechanism to influence and alter the state of mind, which in turn will influence the state of the body and the perception of this physical reality. The habitual nature of the mind, through the subconscious, can be altered towards a balanced harmonious position together with behaviour. The state of the focal and subconscious mind acts as a spotlight on specific frequencies it is aligned to; anger begets more anger and love begets more love, it is the universal law of attraction. The familiarity of a thought will make it much easier to notice and materialise on the outside.

True meditation is to centre one's consciousness in silence, not to go anywhere, or reach for anything, just to be centred in silence. From this position of oneness, prayer and positive affirmations can be introduced for maximum effect.

"Be still and know that I am" - Psalms 46:10

"Meditate in your heart upon your bed and be still" - Psalm 4:4 (AMP)

Meditation is just sitting quietly, whereas prayer is a projection of the consciousness in an affirming way. So to create the right environment for prayer to be effective it must always begin by centering oneself through the act of meditation.

"There is nothing mind can do that cannot be better done in the mind's immobility and thought-free stillness. When mind is still, then truth gets her chance to be heard in the purity of the silence." - Sri Aurobindo

"Meditation is silence. If you realize that you really know nothing, then you will be truly meditating. Such truthfulness is the right soil for silence. Silence is meditation." - Yogaswami

Quotes on meditation:

"Spiritual meditation is the pathway to divinity. It is a mystic ladder which reaches from earth to heaven, from error to truth, from pain to peace." - James Allen

"Meditation is the golden key to all the mysteries of life." - Bhagwan Shree Rajneesh

"Meditation is not something that should be done in a particular position at a particular time. It is an awareness and an attitude that must persist throughout the day." - Annamalai Swami

"Meditation is the dissolution of thoughts in eternal awareness or pure consciousness without objectification, knowing without thinking, merging finitude in infinity." - Sivananda Saraswati

"If you can't meditate in a boiler room, you can't meditate." - Alan Watts

"Meditation, perhaps, is the only alchemy that can transform a beggar into an emperor." - Bhagwan Shree Rajneesh

"Meditation is not a way of making your mind quiet. It is a way of entering into the quiet that is already there—buried under the 50,000 thoughts the average person thinks every day." - Deepak Chopra

Moon cycles and phases

From our earthly perspective the Moon is the fastest moving of all the planets and luminaries. It rotates around the Earth every 27.3 days, this is known as a sidereal month, but because the Earth is also rotating around the Sun, the orbit of the Moon in relation to the position of the Sun takes an extra 2 days, this is referred to as a synodic month of 29.5 days. Each day the Moon moves 12.2 degrees eastwards, occupying each zodiac house for 2.5 days. The Moon produces no light of its own, only reflecting what comes towards it from the Sun, and as it moves around the Earth we experience the Moon's phases, from the new moon, conjunct with the Sun, to a full moon, fully illuminated, opposing the Sun.

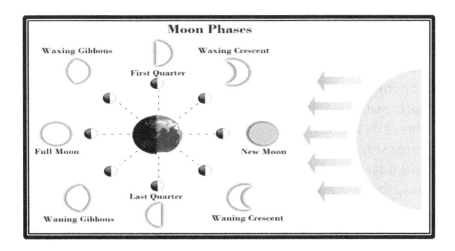

As our perception of reality is a construct within human consciousness, stimulated by our thoughts and planetary bodies, especially the Moon, Its natural cycles and rhythms are therefore important to us when relating to all things to do with our internal subconscious and our spiritual connection to the universe.

The Moon has an influence on the waters of the Earth, and on the monthly cycle of female fertility, it is therefore not unreasonable to expect those influences to continue throughout the waters of the body and the inner mind. With the focal consciousness being only 30% of our minds capacity, it is reasonable to assume that the Moon's connection to our subconscious plays a role in influencing the larger elephantine part of the mind. It is also necessary to comprehend the importance of Moon cycles as they interact with the houses and signs of the zodiac.

Each month there is a new moon, which takes place in a different sign and house of the zodiac. That house should therefore become the backdrop for sowing new seeds within the subconscious and your internal Garden of Eden. The new moon is the start of a new cycle, it is nature's way of initiating a new beginning, or at least an opportunity to tweak that area of life associated with that house which the new moon falls in. Those 2.5 days of the new moon, can be used to plant new positive seeds of intention, dreams and aspirations; a window of opportunity enabling us to communicate with our subconscious elephant. This is the time when meditation can achieve its greatest impact towards reprogramming the subconscious, and altering our perception of reality. Not only can we target those areas of life associated with the specific house the new moon falls in, but also those characteristics synonymous with the houses ruling planet, for example Jupiter would be optimism, abundance and good fortune.

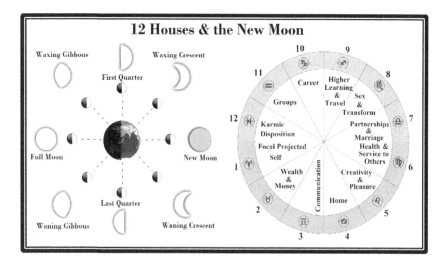

A new moon in Aries (I am), ruled by Mars (proactive energy), would influence Cardinal fire, 1st house of the self, and the focal projected consciousness. During the 2.5 days of this new moon, it is a good time to initiate new beliefs about how you project yourself and come across to others, and how your ego is defined. You could take this opportunity to humble the ego or even encourage it to become more confident. This is all about you, the (I, me, mine). It is also about the head, so anything to do with the head can be brought into the picture, even healing to the head or what ever part of the body is associated with the house each new moon falls in.

To narrow down the zodiac house which is being activated by the new moon, specifically for you, the natives ascendant or rising sign must be taken into account, in order to adjust the house position coming into play. For example, if we have a new moon in Aries, it would influence the first house for rising Arians only, and the second house for rising Taureans, the third house for rising Geminis, the fourth for Cancerians, and so on. Although the new moon's energetic influence, at source, is consistent, it will effect different areas of life depending upon which Moon and rising sign we are born under.

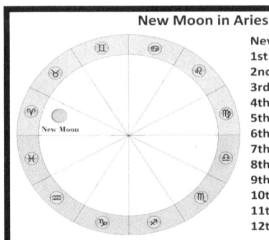

New Moon in Aries

New Moon in Aries
1st House for Aries
2nd House for Taurus
3rd House for Gemini
4th House for Cancer
5th House for Leo
6th House for Virgo
7th House for Libra
8th House for Scorpio
9th House for Sagittarius
10th House for Capricorn
11th House for Aquarius
12th House for Pisces

If an individual has aspirations of becoming a great communicator or of improving his communication skills then instead of placing all of his attention on this goal from a physical perspective, relying solely on that 30% of the mind, which is the focal consciousness; it may be beneficial for him to consider utilising the 70% part of the mind which is commonly dismissed. It may be advantageous to meditate during a new moon in Gemini, and for those 2.5 days of the new moon, all effort should be placed on reprogramming the subconscious, using an array of techniques designed to stimulate the elephant and the Ganesha. With this in mind unwanted obstacles can be removed in order to promote a new internal belief system and path towards better communication and thus a preferably better perception of reality.

If we compare the natural cycle of the female menstrual period with that of the Moon's phases, in relation to developing subconscious reprogramming, we may get closer to understanding the natural process which may take place in order to discard old beliefs in favour of new ones.

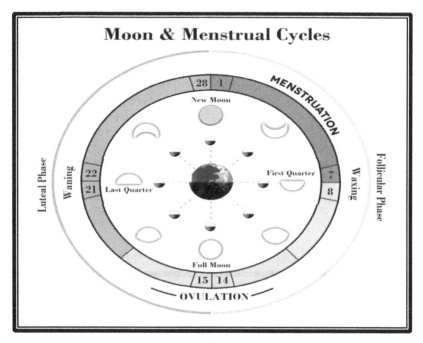

The Start of the menstrual cycle can be compared to the start of a Moon cycle, with the appearance of a new moon every 29.5 days. This can be utilised to discard unwanted subconscious beliefs from the mind. Just as the uterus discharges blood and mucosal tissue from the inner lining during the first seven days of its cycle, this time can be used to create new positive intentions, affirmations and visualisations, helping to sow new seeds and discard old ones. If one persists with regular repetitive reprogramming techniques, the new seeds should germinate. Just as a new egg is produced around 14 days, the full moon should help to bring forth those new subconscious seeds into the physical realm.

Being in tune with nature's cycles is important. Modern living, with its artificial lighting, timing and electro magnetic pollution, is distorting our human biological connection to nature's rhythms, thus pulling us further away from independent self-sufficiency and into the hands of the modern world of globalisation and materialistic interdependency. We have deviated so far away from nature's cycles that modern science doesn't see any relation between the monthly female menstrual cycle and the Moon's orbit of the Earth.

The Lunar effect

In 2007 an article appeared in the Guardian newspaper reporting that Sussex Police were increasing the number of officers deployed in Brighton, due to trouble expected in respect to lunar cycles. A spokeswoman from Sussex police was purported to have said:

"Research carried out by us has shown a correlation between violent incidents and full moons." - The Guardian[2]

The article also goes on to say that a three month psychological study was carried out on 1,200 inmates at

Armley prison in Leeds, in which they found a rise in violent incidents on and around the days of the full moon. This certainly lives up to ideas founded in folklore about full moons and lunacy.

Moon phases effect the gravitational pull of the waters on the Earth, when the Moon is in syzygy (in a straight line) with the Sun and the Earth, the greatest tide extremes are produced. This is also thought to have an effect on soil moisture and plant life, along with light variations, giving rise to the art of planting by Moon phases. It has been suggested that crops which grow above ground prefer the waxing phase, while root crops prefer the waning phase, the area associated with the lower part of the zodiac and the root chakra.

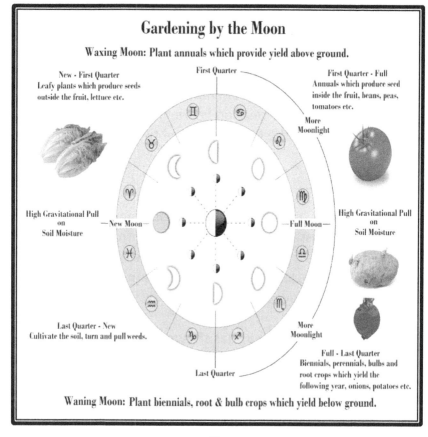

Gardening by the Moon

Waxing Moon: Plant annuals which provide yield above ground.

New - First Quarter
Leafy plants which produce seeds outside the fruit, lettuce etc.

First Quarter

First Quarter - Full
Annuals which produce seed inside the fruit, beans, peas, tomatoes etc.

More Moonlight

High Gravitational Pull on Soil Moisture — New Moon —

— Full Moon — High Gravitational Pull on Soil Moisture

More Moonlight

Last Quarter - New
Cultivate the soil, turn and pull weeds.

Last Quarter

Full - Last Quarter
Biennials, perennials, bulbs and root crops which yield the following year, onions, potatoes etc.

Waning Moon: Plant biennials, root & bulb crops which yield below ground.

"The old-time gardeners say, "With the waxing of the Moon, the earth exhales. When the sap in the plants rise, the force first goes into the growth above ground. Thus, you should do all activities with plants that bear fruit above ground during a waxing moon. With the waning of the Moon, the earth inhales. Then, the sap primarily goes down toward the roots. Thus, the waning moon is a good time for pruning, multiplying, fertilizing, watering, harvesting, and controlling parasites and weeds"" - Ute York, Living by the Moon.[3]

"Increasing amount of moonlight stimulates leaf growth, and as the moonlight decreases the above ground leaf growth slows down. The root is stimulated again." - John Jeavons. How to grow more vegetables.[4]

It is quite obvious that the Moon has a huge impact on the waters in the physical realm, but because the material world of modern science does not acknowledge the spiritual realm, including metaphysics, it dismisses any possible internal effect or interaction between the Moon and the subconscious. Therefore, subconscious reprogramming with the aid of Moon phases, is not something which will be considered as a plausible remedy when trying to help people. The sales and consumption of antidepressants is preferred, by the drug industrial complex, as a long term treatment for subconscious and focal mind disharmony.

Unfortunately most western and modern societies have been socially engineered with a rigid belief that the individual has no power of their own, and that they must look outside themselves, towards the state, and its many organised institutions, for remedies to all the ills which a person may face throughout their lives. From a very early age most people are conditioned to believe only in the physical realm, and that the subconscious is not something they should be concerned about, the elephant has been given its instructions, in those

42

formative early years, and it is not necessary to interfere any further; just keep on working, consuming and drinking, the elephant should be ignored and left to its own devices.

The Moon is all about internal needs, it is emotional sensitivity and requires emotional fulfillment on a deep internal and spiritual level. It is sometimes regarded as the PAC-MAN due to its need for internal fulfillment. Consequently, it holds the key to our habitual nature along with eating habits. The word mood is derived from the Moon, as the fastest and closest moving planetary body in the heavens, its transits have a deep emotional and spiritual influence on our biology and perception of reality. The German word for mood is 'laune', another connection to the Moon or Luna. Moreover, because the Moon moves through the signs and houses relatively quickly, our moods change with the angle of Lunar transits as they interact with the position of our natal planets, challenging our karmic disposition. Occasionally when the Moon's transiting angle or Arch-angel Gabriel comes up against hard inharmonious angles with other planet and signs it is referred to as a 'bad moon rising'.

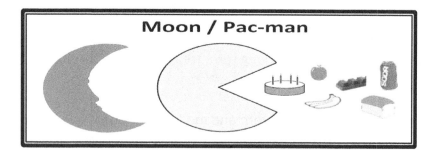

Cancer

The choice and use of the word 'cancer' to describe a dis-ease, which from a metaphysical perspective is the result of an imbalance within the body's internal mechanisms of well being, harmony and subconscious chi energy, seems more than just a coincidence. Cancer is of course the zodiac sign ruled by the Moon, represented by the crab, which was known in ancient Greek as 'cancer'. The accepted reason for this choice of the word, described in medical literature, is due to the cancerous tumor having a similar appearance to the legs of a crab.

Hippocrates 460-370bc considered to be the father of medicine, used the terms carcinos and carcinoma to describe non-ulcer forming and ulcer forming tumors. In Greek these words refer to a crab. Projections from a cancer look like a crab.[5]

From a metaphysical perspective, when our internal spirit and karmic disposition becomes in-harmoniously detached from the physical soul, the result can promote dis-ease within the biological framework of the body. The further that soul and spirit detachment, together with a disregard for nature's rhythms and cycles, the greater chance of some form of physical response to this predicament. Cancer, the 4th house of the zodiac, is the house concerned with the home, personal needs and feelings of inner security. If this is undermined or infested with stress, there is a chance that the sign of Cancer may precipitate some unwanted manifestations in the physical realm.

Natal charts and planetary influence on weight gain

When analysing a persons birth chart, certain planetary positions and aspects can be interpreted as susceptibility to weight gain. If this is the case, certain measures can be introduced to counter this natural disposition. There are many variations and interpretations to this depending upon who is reading the birth chart and the criteria they have adopted. But to keep it simple we shall concentrate on just a few planets, the Moon for internal needs, Jupiter for expansion /

abundance, Venus for sugar and Mars for proactive physical energy relating to metabolism.

Each planet's unique characteristics has the potential to influence us both positively and negatively. This could be viewed as a virtue or a vice. Too much unrestrained Jupiter energy can result in its vice 'gluttony' being expressed in a persons eating habits, Saturn also has a vice, with the potential to promote greed. Consequently, the position of certain planets either in the birth chart or in day to day transits can promote unwanted vices in one's life.

Virtues or Vices		
Planet	Virtue	Vice
Sun	Humility (humbleness)	Pride (vanity)
Moon	Diligence (zeal/integrity/labor)	Sloth (laziness/idleness)
Mars	Forgiveness (composure)	Wrath (anger)
Mercury	Kindness (admiration)	Envy (jealousy)
Jupiter	Temperance (self-restraint)	Gluttony (over-indulgence)
Venus	Chastity (purity)	Lust (excessive sexual appetites)
Saturn	Charity (giving)	Greed (avarice)

Jupiter

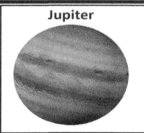

Planet of expansion, abundance, good fortune, hope, optimism and good will.

Vice = Gluttony

Takes 12 years to orbit the Sun, stays in each house for 1 year.

$$\frac{\text{Crescent of spirituality}}{\text{Cross of physical body}}$$

Venus

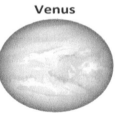

Planet of love, liking and all things sweet. Known as 'Shukra' in Sanskrit, and is where the word sugar originates.

Vice = Lust

Takes 225 days to orbit the Sun, staying in each house for 18 days.

$$\frac{\text{Focal consciousness}}{\text{Physical body}}$$

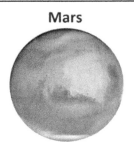

Mars

Planet of proactive physical energy.

Vice = Anger

Takes 687 days to orbit the Sun, stays in each house for 57 days.

$$\frac{\text{Physical movement in a direction}}{\text{Focal consciousness}}$$

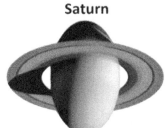

Saturn

Planet of restriction, pessimism, loss, order and control.

Vice = Greed

Takes 29.4 years to orbit the Sun, stays in each house for 2.5 days.

$$\frac{\text{Cross of physical body}}{\text{Crescent of spirituality}}$$

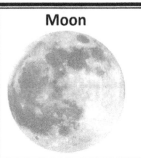

Moon

Planet of the subconscious, internal emotions, needs and habitual nature.

Vice = Laziness

Synodic month is 29.5 days, staying in each house 2.5 days.

Spirit / Subconscious

In my first book *'Language of the Gods'* I explain, in detail, how each monotheistic religion has singled out one planet over all the others to represent their overall characteristics and philosophy. Christianity promotes Jupiterian optimism, Islam promotes Venus, Buddhism promotes Mercury and Judaism promotes and aligns itself with the energetic characteristics of Saturn. This simple underlining observation explains the many differences expressed in various cultures that have adopted these religions. For example Jupiter is the planet of abundance and expansion, it is the largest planet in our solar system, and as such, reflects these characteristics throughout the Christian world. Jupiter was known as Zeus in ancient Greece and through their adopted ambassador Jupiter/Zeus (Juzeus) all the expansive, goodwill and good fortune characteristics have heavily influenced the followers of the Christian faith. As Jupiter is the largest and most expansive planet in the solar system, it was no coincidence to see Christianity become the largest and most expansive religion in the world, especially during the Age of Pisces.

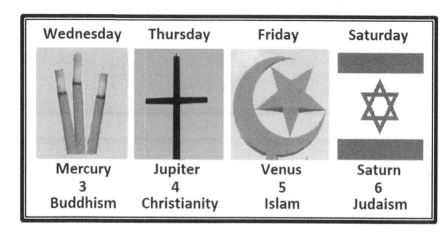

Wednesday	Thursday	Friday	Saturday
Mercury	Jupiter	Venus	Saturn
3	4	5	6
Buddhism	Christianity	Islam	Judaism

A recent study for the Journal of Religion and Health, found that Christians are more likely to have a larger BMI (body mass index) than atheists and other religious groups.

"Evidence of this association was strongest among those affiliated to a Christian religion" Dr Deborah Lycett, a senior lecturer in dietetics at Coventry University.[6]

Moreover, the word for the planet Mercury in Sanskrit is 'Budha'. Muslims pray five times a day and adhere to the five pillars of Islam, and Judaism is synonymous with the number 6, Saturn and the Sabbath.

With this in mind, we can assume that the relative position of certain planets in a persons birth chart and /or their religious allegiance to certain planetary energies can have an influence on their overall body weight. With the Moon being the planet associated with internal habitual needs and Jupiter being the planet of abundance and expansion, we can look for correlations with these planetary positions and transits in those people who are seriously overweight.

To appreciate how these planetary influences play out in one's life, it is necessary to understand the ascendant and the area of the natal chart which reflects an individuals personal identity. While the first house, in a person's chart, relates to the projected self and focal consciousness, the twelfth house is the subconscious and karmic disposition. The first house, twelfth house and ascendant are all part of our personal identity, which can be viewed as a stage, where the first house is the front of the stage; the twelfth house is the enormous back stage along with dressing rooms; and the ascendant can be seen as those first impressions, the moment we walk out on the stage.

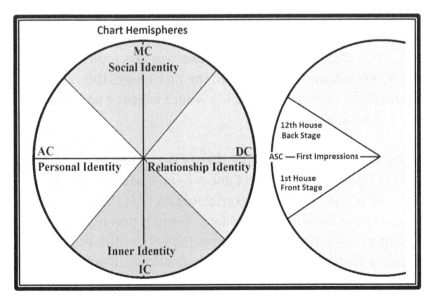

The square is the most dynamic aspect, at 90 degrees, it creates strong electromagnetic torque which generates tension between the planets and their relative chart positions, promoting action in order to resolve external pressures or internal conflicts.

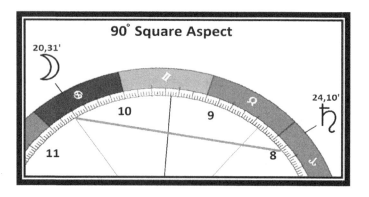

Although all the planets have the potential to promote excessive weight gain, certain planets like Jupiter, when either conjunct (together) or in conflict (square 90 degrees) with a persons ascendant, will focus Jupiter's expansive gluttonous potential towards an individual's personal identity. Likewise, as Jupiter transits (moves) around the chart, over the course of a person's lifetime, occasionally creates hard squaring aspects to the ascendant, giving rise to some periods of expansion due to gluttony. Every twelve years Jupiter transits the ascendant and goes through the first house, this is regarded as a period in one's life where weight gain has a good chance of occurring.

Many astrologers support the theory that if Jupiter is found in watery signs like Pisces and Cancer (water being synonymous with the Moon and the subconscious) there is the potential for excessive weight gain. Similarly, there is potential for weight gain if Jupiter is badly aspected with either the Sun (focal consciousness) or Moon (subconscious). Below are a few examples:

Oliver Hardy's birth chart
18 January 1892, 9:02 AM, Atlanta, Georgia (US)

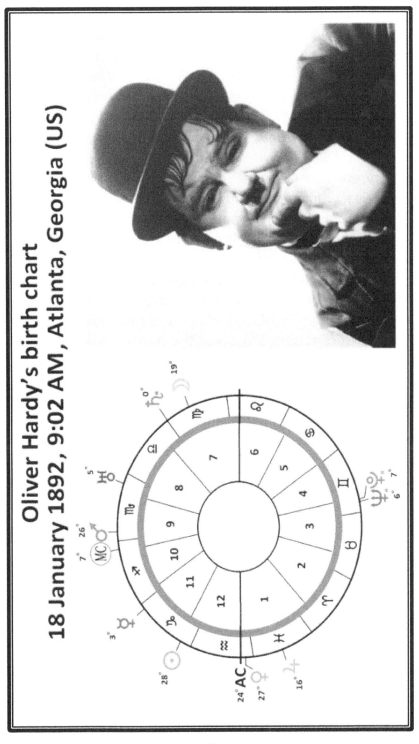

Oliver Hardy's birth chart is interesting in a variety of ways, regarding his weight. Jupiter (I expand) is positioned in his first house of the projected self, which also happens to be in Pisces, one of the gluttonous water signs. We also find Venus in the first house, close to the ascendant. In Sanskrit Venus was known as 'Shukra', it is the planet of all things sweet, and the origin of our word 'sugar'. This Jupitarian abundance of all things sweet would have manifested in Hardy's personal identity, and how he was seen to the outside world. Every twelve years Jupiter's transiting return would have also played a role in promoting times of over indulgence and gluttony. Which ever planet transits through his ascendant will shower its influence over his personal identity, promoting variations to his general behaviour. While Jupiter is known for expanding a person's weight, Saturn can influence us in the opposite way. Saturn is an inversion of Jupiter's, crescent over the cross, characteristics, it is the cross over the crescent, associated with restriction, loss and control. Saturn is the slowest of the traditional planets seen with the naked eye, consequently, it was known as 'Old Father Time'. When Saturn passes the ascendant it can promote weight loss along with improved control over one's projected self and personal identity. Mars, the planet of proactive energy can stimulate the metabolism into burning off excessive fat. Venus will promote cravings for all things sweet, especially when conjunct with the pacman Moon (I need) as it moves close towards the ascendant.

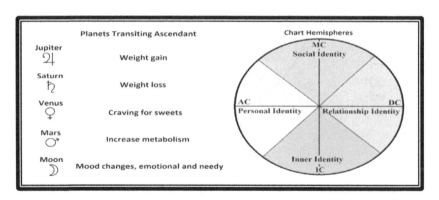

Natal Sun and Moon

Along with the ascendant, the position of one's natal Sun and Moon will also play a part with transiting planets throughout the course of a person's life. The Sun being associated with the focal consciousness will draw your attention to any extra influence offered by transiting planets like Jupiter. When Jupiter conjuncts the natal Sun it stimulates its characteristics and expansive tendencies within one's physical reality and wants. The natal Moon, being associated with the greater part of the mind, the subconscious, will also be effected by transiting planets, influencing emotional needs deep within our habitual nature. A good example of this can be seen in Elvis Presley's birth chart together with the transiting influence of Jupiter on his natal Sun and Moon, in the final years of his life. Elvis Presley ballooned during the 1970s, contributing to his death in 1977.

As can be seen from Elvis's birth chart, he has Jupiter on his personal identity side of his chart, near the ascendant, in the water sign of Scorpio (I desire), combining to create 'I desire to expand.' What is important here is the transit dates of Jupiter as it interacts with his natal ascendant, Sun and Moon. Every twelve years Jupiter moves a full cycle around the chart, heavily influencing Elvis to expand even more. During the first two Jupiter returns Elvis was a young man with a high metabolic rate, especially while he was working. The problem came on Jupiter's 3rd return in 1972, as Jupiter crosses his ascendant he was 37 years old and his metabolism was slowing down. Instead of cutting back on the calories and carbohydrates he became gluttonous, consuming thousands of calories per day. In 1973 Jupiter conjuncts his natal Sun promoting his focal consciousness to home in on expansion and gluttony, passing Venus the sugar planet for bouts and cravings for all things sweet. In 1975 Jupiter's transit homes in on Elvis's natal Moon, setting in motion gluttonous habitual

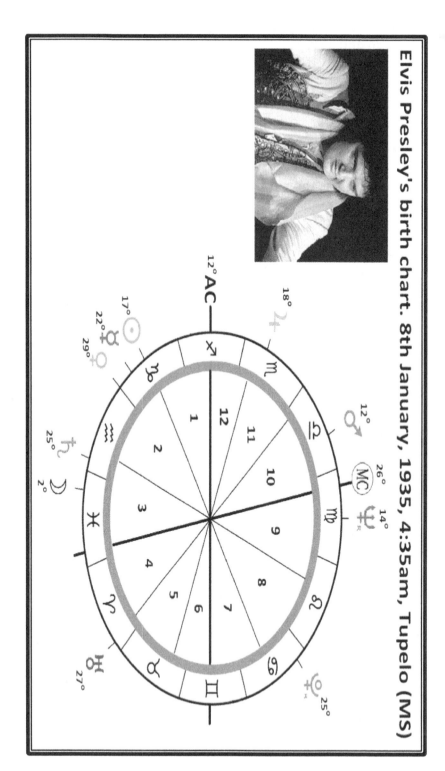

Elvis Presley's birth chart. 8th January, 1935, 4:35am, Tupelo (MS)

needs within the powerful mind of the subconscious. This is the point of no return for Elvis, according to some sources , by the time of his death in 1977, he was consuming a whopping 10-12,000 calories per day. He had expanded to 159kg or 25 stone.[7] This is a great example of how vulnerable the subconscious is to unhealthy habits, and as we grow older we must take control over what seeds we allow to germinate within its garden. Although planetary influences are there, they are subtle and no match for an individual's will power in overriding their unwanted potential. What you focus your attention on is ultimately the source of the seeds which may or may not germinate into new habits.

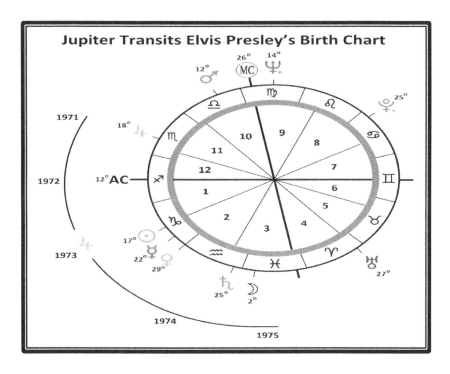

Jupiter Transits Elvis Presley's Birth Chart

Mars is also important when looking at weight gain, as it is a planet associated with proactive energy and the metabolism. A good aspected Mars can promote calorie burn, whereas a bad aspected Mars will do the opposite. When Mars goes retrograde (appearing to move backwards from our earthly perspective) it is considered to be a time when weight gain is highly probable. This is because, when the planet of proactive energy and physical movement goes retrograde it is thought to have a detrimental effect on a person's metabolism. There are so many factors to consider when analysing a birth chart, together with daily transits, that it takes an experienced chart reader to interpret what cosmic energies are at play at any given time.

Appetite and cravings

Throughout our lives our weight, appetite and energy levels fluctuate. From an astrological perspective this could well be the result of cosmic cycles having an influence on our biology. The Moon's phases play a significant role in our internal needs and emotions and are thought to influence not only our moods but also our cravings for food.

New Moon

- Increased appetite.
- Emotional energy increased.
- Increase in intuition and new ideas.
- More deeper sleep.
- Clear insight.
- Feel more introverted, sensitive and detached.

Full Moon (reflects a maximum of 12% of the Sun's light)

- Decreased appetite.
- Physical energy increased.
- More wants as opposed to needs.
- Sexuality is at a peak.
- More likely to stay out late.
- Dreams come into focal awareness.

Notes for chapter 2

(1) Teal Swan. Using orgasm to replace painful beliefs, tealswan.com, 2018.
https://tealswan.com/resources/articles/using-orgasm-to-repl ace-painful-beliefs-r215/

(2) Fred Attewell, Police link full moon to aggression, The Guardian, 5th June 2007,
https://www.theguardian.com/uk/2007/jun/05/ukcrime

(3) Ute York, Living by the Moon, Published by Bluestar Communication Corp, Woodside, California, U.S.A., 1997,
https://www.abebooks.co.uk/Living-Moon-Practical-Guide-Ch oosing-Right/11206846310/bd

(4) John Jeavons, How to grow more vegetables, Ten Speed Press; 8 edition (February 7, 2012),
https://www.amazon.com/How-Grow-More-Vegetables-Eight h/dp/160774189X

(5) The American Cancer Society Medical and Editorial Content Team, Early History of Cancer, Defining Cancer, 2014.
https://www.cancer.org/cancer/cancer-basics/history-of-canc er/what-is-cancer.html

(6) Lianna Brinded, Christians are more likely to be fat than atheists, December 2014, International Business Times,
http://www.ibtimes.co.uk/christians-are-more-likely-be-fat-at heists-1480732

(7) Rachel Hosie, Elvis Presley's diet, The Independent, August 2017,
https://www.independent.co.uk/life-style/food-and-drink/elvi s-presley-diet-how-lose-weight-king-what-eat-normal-day-me als-peanut-butter-sandwich-a7896076.html

Chapter 3. The metaphysical diet

The basic principle of this diet is to harmonise with nature's cycles. We are, after all, biological expressions of consciousness living within the constraints of time and space, upon an earth of abundant natural beauty and cosmic cycles. As such, the more in tune we are with these timeless natural rhythms and planetary cycles the less chance we have of falling into dis-harmony and dis-ease.

Nature expresses itself through the number 12, it is the universal number of harmony, balance and completion. It was a numerical benchmark for most of our ancestors and those who lived in ancient civilisations. It can be found in the following:

The Number 12	
12 hours on the clock face.	12 tribes of Israel.
12 months of the year.	12 grades at school.
12 signs and houses of the zodiac.	12 members of a jury.
12 notes in a musical scale.	12 cranial nerves.
12 inches in a foot.	12 pairs of ribs.
12 pennies to 1 imperial shilling.	12 pints of blood in an adult
12 Apostles.	12% of sunlight reflected from full Moon

Our ancestors, such as the Romans and the Greeks generally lived within the confines of daylight hours. They would wake up at dawn, when the Sun appeared on the horizon, and perform most of their daily routine between the hours of 6am and 6pm, and then retire for the evening. Once the Sun went down only the wealthy could afford artificial lighting, subjecting the vast majority to an early night of rest and sleep. Preparing or cooking food during evening hours came with a variety of problems, consequently, most people at this time in history would eat one meal a day (OMAD), which was consumed in the middle of the daylight hours, between 12 noon and 2pm.

"The Romans typically only ate 1 meal a day and did so around noon time. This was not only to hold them over to complete their daily tasks, but it was truly the only food they had available for the course of the day as well. The Roman culture actually believed it to be far healthier to eat only 1 meal a day." - Omaddiet.com[1]

As astrology is the oldest living language known to man, a language which expresses our human conscious connection and relationship to nature, the macrocosm and planetary cycles, it was used by many ancient cultures as the benchmark for most of their activities. If we look at the first six houses of the zodiac during the daylight hours, we find the house ruled by the Moon, our internal needs or hungry pacman, is in Cancer between 12 noon and 2pm.

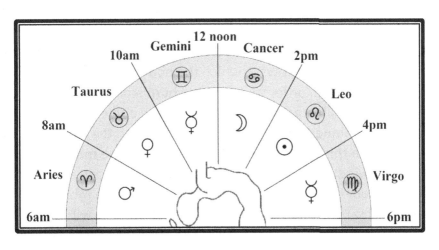

By restricting yourself to only eating during this time, essentially having one meal a day, you can eat, within reason, most of the things you enjoy, and as much as you like, to satisfy your basic feelings of hunger. People who have lost control of their eating habits need to take back the reins and steer themselves towards sensible eating patterns. It is important not to overeat, as it unnecessarily expands the stomach, sending you back towards your old unhealthy ways. You are the only one who can change course, by reprogramming your subconscious elephant into accepting new behavioral patterns. The overall objective is to be the greatest version of yourself at this moment in time, optimistically setting the sails for a brighter future.

Intermittent fasting and breaking the fast

The zodiac's poetical synchronicity is profound in many ways, and those who use it as a guide to support their lives can appreciate its esoteric wisdom and worth. By eliminating the consumption of food in the morning, you essentially extend the fasting process which began a few hours after you ate the previous day's meal. The time the fast is broken (break-fast) is crucial to the success of the metaphysical diet. It must be in tune with nature, allowing enough time for the body to use up its store of calories consumed by the previous meal. By only eating during the 2 hour window between noon and 2pm, a process of fasting follows in which the body changes its hormone levels in order to utilise and burn stored energy which is deposited as fat in cells all over the body. This fasting process continues for 22 hours until it is broken the following noon. Once this is accepted as a new daily routine many benefits will start to take place concerning your body and your health. Your stomach will shrink to a point where a modest meal will satisfy, and you will gradually lose weight without too much discomfort. Those old habits which are killing you have to be neutralised and removed. The first week of any challenge to old habits is always the most difficult, just like the female menstrual (moonstrual) cycle it begins with shedding of unwanted matter from a previous cycle. You must do the same and persevere with will power alone until this new habit is accepted within the corridors of the subconscious.

Many things happen when we fast:[2]

- Insulin levels drop to facilitate the fat burning process.
- Human growth hormone increases by up to five times stimulating fat burn.
- The body's natural cellular repair process increases together with the removal of waste material from the cells.
- Testosterone levels increase and estrogen levels decrease, which promotes fat burn.
- Intermittent fasting can increase metabolic rate by up to 14%.

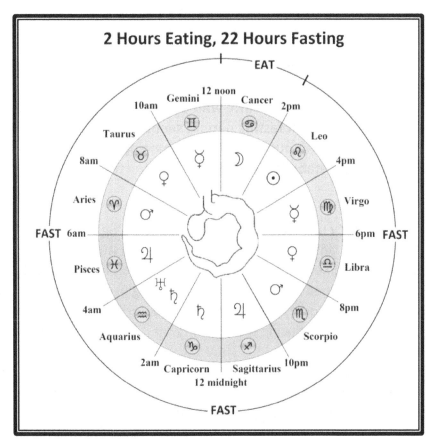

Studies have shown that periodic and intermittent fasting can reduce the aging process and increase your life span by a considerable amount. A recent Harvard University study found that fasting can increase lifespan and slow down the aging process by stimulating mitochondrial networks inside cells.

"Although previous work has shown how intermittent fasting can slow aging, we are only beginning to understand the underlying biology," - "Our findings open up new avenues in the search for therapeutic strategies that will reduce our likelihood of developing age-related diseases as we get older." - William Mair[3]

Scientists at the (NIA) National Institute on Aging at the University of Wisconsin-Madison, and the Pennington Biomedical Research Center, Baton Rouge, Louisiana, conducted a study on mice, where they found increased fasting times led to improved health and longevity.

"This study showed that mice who ate one meal per day, and thus had the longest fasting period, seemed to have a longer lifespan and better outcomes for common age-related liver disease and metabolic disorders," - NIA Director Richard J. Hodes, M.D.[4]

Another study undertaken by evolutionary biologist Dr Margo Adler, at the University of New South Wales in Australia, concerning the effects of dietary restrictions on human health, concluded that eating less can benefit the aging process by protecting the body's cells from natural deterioration, with the potential of reducing the risk of cancer, she went on to say:

"This is the most intriguing aspect from a human health standpoint. Although extended lifespan may simply be a side effect of dietary restriction, a better understanding of these

cellular recycling mechanisms that drive the effect may hold the promise of longer, healthier lives for humans." - Dr Margo Adler[5]

In order to make the diet agreeable and practical the intake of fluids is not restricted throughout the whole day. You can basically drink as much as you want as long as the drinks throughout the morning period do not contain sugar or milk, this is because your blood sugar level and insulin must be kept low for fat burn to continue. As a basic guideline stick to water or black tea and coffee. With water being 70% of the body's composition, and synonymous with the Moon and the subconscious, it is important to consume ample quantities in order to keep the body and mind hydrated. The common consensus among many health authorities is an intake of 2 liters of water per day, the benefits of which include:

● Water maintains the correct balance of body fluids.
● By drinking water you are not increasing your calorie intake.
● Muscle cells work well when the body is completely hydrated.
● Helps to keep the skin in good condition.
● Keeps the kidneys flushed, working well to remove toxins.
● Balanced the hydration on the colon preventing constipation.

Religious fasting

Most religions practice some form of fasting, a tradition which goes back a very long way. Many believed the eating process, especially meats, would toxify the body during digestion disrupting the body's natural balance between body, soul and spirit. In times of high spiritual significance, it was considered necessary to keep the body's chemical equilibrium clean for greatest metaphysical impact.

Fasting in Christianity

Although modern Christianity has splintered off into a multitude of perversions, deviating from the source of its heritage, some serious Christians still practice the art of fasting, mainly during the 40 days of Lent. Many religious festivals are based around important zodiacal transitions, although they do not like to admit it. The 40 days of Lent takes place during the Spring Equinox, bringing in the start of a new zodiac cycle. Today only a small minority of Christians fast during this period, usually restricting their eating to the night time, many refrain from eating meat, those who do fast generally do it on Ash Wednesday and Good Friday as a gesture of respect for their God.

Fasting in Buddhism

Buddhism is an ancient religion/philosophy. It goes back 2500 years to the time of Gautama Buddha, a sage who from the age of 29 left his rich and privileged home to find wisdom and enlightenment. Budha with one 'd' is Sanskrit for the planet Mercury, the planet of communication. Its energetic characteristics are necessary for good communication between all levels of consciousness.

The monks which follow Buddhism are essentially Moon watches, they are moonks. Buddha understood the importance of fasting and said to his followers:

"I, monks, do not eat a meal in the evening. Not eating a meal in the evening. I, monks, am aware of good health and of being without illness and of buoyancy and strength and living in comfort. Come, do you too, monks, not eat a meal in the evening. Not eating a meal in the evening you too, monks, will be aware of good health and..... living in comfort." - Gautama Buddha

Buddhist monks follow the Vinaya (discipline, education), they are allowed to eat from dawn till mid-day. However, Buddha did recommend his followers to only eat one meal per day to promote good health and stimulate the meditation process.

"Buddha encouraged monks to have one meal per day as that is good for health and helps in the meditation practice. It is also part of the 13 ascetic practices (Dhutanga) which is voluntarily taken up as part of the practice." - Dhammagavesi Bhikkhu[6]

Fasting is part of a lay Buddhists life, during times of intensive meditation, especially during the four main phases of the moon, the monks avoid eating animal products. Furthermore, they also avoid eating processed foods along with the five pungent foods: garlic, welsh onion, garlic, chives, asana and leeks.[7]

Fasting in Islam

The main period for fasting for Muslims is during the month of Ramadan. It is the 9th month of the Islamic lunar calendar. This year, 2018, it took place from 17th May to 14th June. Muslims believe that fasting helps develop good behaviour, self control and purifies the connection between body and soul. Together with their fasting they incorporate abstinence from any falsehoods, either in speech or action. They refrain from cursing, arguing, fighting, ignorant speech together with disassociating themselves from lustful thoughts.

"This purification of body and soul harmonizes the inner and outer spheres of an individual. Muslims aim to improve their body by reducing food intake and maintaining a healthier lifestyle." - Fasting in Islam, Wikipedia.

All Muslims are expected to participate in Ramadan, fasting for one whole month, beginning at sunrise and ending at sunset.

Fasting in Judaism

As Judaism is a religion which promotes the planet Saturn above all others, a planet synonymous with the black cube and the number six. It is therefore understandable to find they traditionally fast for only six days of the year. On a fasting day they abstain from both food and drink. However, fasting is not permitted on the Sabbath, Saturday (Saturn's day), unless it happens to coincide with Yom Kippur, the most important holy day in the Jewish calendar. Being the only fast day mentioned in the Torah, all Jews above the age of bat mitzvah (12-13) are expected to fast on Yom Kippur (2018 was 18-19th September).

Another fasting day for Jews is Tisha B'av (2018 was 21-22nd July). This is a significant day in Jewish history, where a number of disasters occurred, for instance, the destruction of Solomon's Temple. Jewish fasting takes place between sunset of one day to dusk of the next. Dusk normally takes place around half an hour after sunset.

Fasting in Hinduism

Due to the enormous number of different Gods worshipped by Hindus, along with the many variations in local customs, fasting is more of an individual choice integral within their worshipping process. No food or water is to be consumed from sunset of one day to 48 minutes after sunrise the next. It is also common for Hindus to limit themselves to one meal during the day, restricting the variety of foods on offer, especially meat products.

New moon fasting and meditation

Putting all this information together concerning the fasting process, the subconscious, meditation and the Moon, it appears logical to combine all of these important concepts in order to promote healthy eating habits over those which have underpinned many people's weight problems. It is vital that one takes control over their habitual nature, by redirecting their subconscious elephant in a new, healthy and sustainable direction. Because fasting is a great aid in reducing unnecessary toxification from food consumption, giving the body time to re-balance chemically and hormonaly, it seems sensible to promote fasting during the most sensitive Moon phases, in order for the internal subconscious mind to germinate new seeds of positive intent at a time when better communication between body, soul and spirit can be utilised. Because Moon phases are reflected in the female menstrual cycle, the metaphysical diet has been carefully designed to make the most of the new moon, a time when nature offers us the opportunity to sow new seeds of intent within the subconscious. Together with fasting, meditation is recommended as a mechanism of communicating with the internal mind, consequently, the whole day of the new moon should be a day of fasting and meditation, eliminating all food stuffs, allowing only water or natural teas into the body. This prepares the body and generates the necessary platform for successful meditation. Moreover, for the new moon fasting day to be successful, it is better to place yourself in a quiet location with few distractions, making it easier to internalise the mind. As this is a day dedicated to the subconscious, with a new moon, it makes perfect sense to go somewhere quiet like a temple, a church, or in a quiet location by water. The fasting process will naturally help to internalise the mind due to the body's limited energy. If no suitable location is available home is the next best thing, as home is represented by the 4th zodiac house, ruled by the Moon.

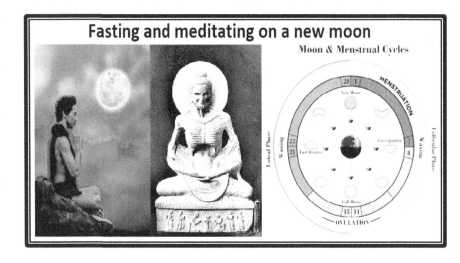

Fasting and meditating on a new moon

Moon & Menstrual Cycles

In addition to the new moon, its placement in relation to an individual's birth chart is also significant. Each month the new moon manifests in a new zodiac house, and each house corresponds to a particular aspect of an individual's personality and life's categories. For example, if the new moon falls in a person's first house, it will stimulate, during this Moon cycle, the projected self within the subconscious. Consequently, to maximize the impact of the opportunity, one's meditation mantra and focus should be relevant to the characteristics of the house the new moon falls in. These relevant house positions are determined by the placing of a person's ascendant. This is calculated by knowing the precise time of birth. If this is not known, the sign In which the new moon falls in becomes the overriding backdrop for the focus on meditation. The ascendant is usually found on the far left of the chart, a point representing the eastern horizon at the moment of birth.

To significantly benefit from the meditation opportunity, as an addition, it is also worth introducing some traditional techniques, which will promote an all round positive outcome to the meditation process. Along with positive affirmations concerning the house the new moon falls in, a good additional technique, as previously mentioned, is to think of three people, one who you love, one who is neutral, and one who you have problems with, even dislike. In turn wish them all well, as you view them in your mind. If this is done on a regular basis, the garden within the subconscious will begin to change, enabling a whole new habitual nature to grow from within.

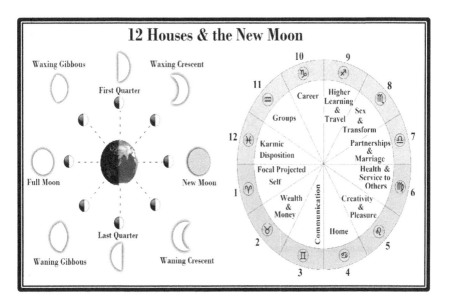

Siesta and exercise

Keeping in tune with nature and following on from the zodiac sign of Cancer, we enter the sign of Leo (the will of a lion), ruled by the Sun, between 2pm and 4pm. Throughout the ancient Mediterranean world, together with many other hot countries, the tradition of taking an afternoon nap became very popular. Many countries still practice a siesta (Spanish for 'nap'), from a combination of drowsiness felt after their afternoon meal, and the unbearable heat during the hottest part of the day, a well deserved break was welcomed. There is an old saying "to sleep like a lion," lions can sleep a great deal, up to 20 hours a day if necessary.[8] Various studies have been carried out which suggest the best time to take an afternoon nap is between 2-3pm.[9] In 2007 the Washington Post reported on a study undertaken in Greece which showed those people who took an afternoon nap greatly reduced their risk of having a heart attack.[10] The reason why this is profoundly interesting is because the body part associated with the sign of Leo is the heart.

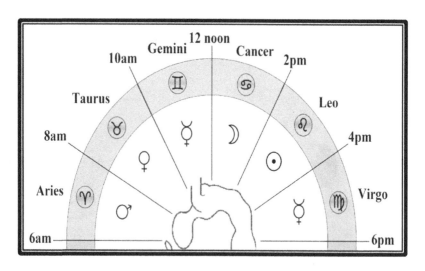

After Leo we move into Virgo, between 4pm and 6pm. This is also the 6th house of health and service to others. Studies have shown that this is the best time for exercise. The overall body temperature increases throughout the day, with heart rate and blood pressure falling, making late afternoon the best time for exercise.[11]

It is also good practice to get the heart pumping and kick-start the day with some form of cardio exercise between 6 and 8am. This is the sign of Aries, ruled by Mars, the planet of proactive physical energy and cardinal fire. 30 minutes is ample, just to get the blood circulating, in preparation for the day ahead. Most people are in a rush to go to work, so whatever you can do in the morning will be of benefit, even if it is just simple exercises in the bedroom, try to do something to increase your heart rate.

When considering the later exercise between 4-6pm, whatever type of exercise you choose, it is important to keep in tune with nature. Consequently, if you are someone who enjoys the gym, it is recommended that repetition of sets are done in twelves, the universal number of harmony, balance and completion. These sets should also be done four times, as four is another important number, both in nature and metaphysically.

- 4 cardinal points (NEWS).
- 4 phases of the Moon.
- 4 is the glyph for Jupiter, the planet of optimism, abundance and good fortune.
- 4 elements (earth, air, fire, water).
- 4 is the house of Cancer in the zodiac ruled by the Moon.
- 4 rivers flow out of Eden.
- 4 nobel truths in Buddhism.
- 4 seasons.

When working out in the Gym, instead of just automatically counting from 1 to 12. It is a golden opportunity to introduce positive mantra, in an effort to influence the subconscious into working towards your latest dreams, wishes and aspirations. Repetition is a simple way of conversing with the subconscious and formulating new internal beliefs. So instead of just counting, it is better to repeat and visualize the words 'I am slim, happy and healthy. By counting in an ascending fashion you automatically generate a comfortable internal belief in expansion and the expectation of a growing sequence. This will ultimately manifest as an expectation of growth in various other areas of life too. One method is to visualize the zodiac as you recite your mantra assigning each word to one of the 12 houses as you go around.

I am slim, happy, healthy
or
I am wealthy, happy, healthy

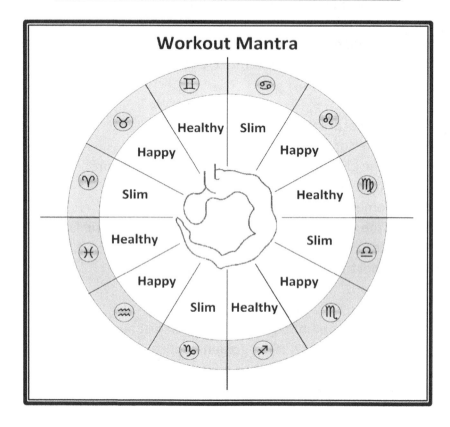

Substitute each word in place of a number, repeating it 4 times to produce 12 repetitions. It is also a good idea to warm up on one of many types of cardio machines for 12 minutes prior to your workout, also ending with 4 minutes, as a final cool down giving you an extra calorie burn opportunity before you leave. It is not necessary to go to the gym or exercise religiously every day. Every other day is good enough to burn off excess fat, improve stamina and generally lift you out of the unhealthy trap which you have fallen into. By going 3 or 4 times a week, you are more likely to look forward to the workouts instead of becoming disillusioned with the monotony related to every day training . Try and keep things fresh and interesting by incorporating new exercises and even different venues.

When significant changes are implemented in a persons life, like the metaphysical diet, it is worth viewing those changes from the perspective of nature and natural cycles. The female menstrual cycle, together with the Moon's phases, give us a good indicator as to what to expect. The first week, of any habit breaking, is always the most difficult, as it is the beginning of a whole new approach to what ever changes we are trying to achieve. Old habits must be discarded, just like the menstruation period in the woman's moonthly cycle. After 2 weeks we see the full moon, the maximum illumination from the Sun, the focal consciousness, bringing forth results of sown seeds into the physical realm. This is also when the egg appears in the female's reproductive system. It is the point at which those new seeds of positive intention start to manifest as new habitual behavioral patterns in the real world.

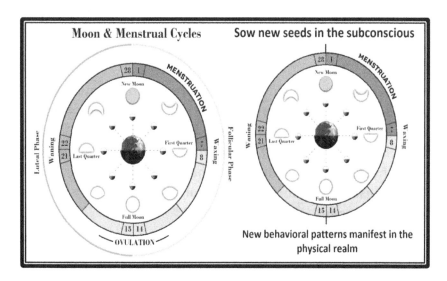

We have moved so far away from nature's cycles that modern science cannot find any connection between lunar rhythms and the female menstrual cycle, concluding that the fact both cycles last 28 days is just a mere coincidence.[12] They fail to appreciate the impact Moon cycles have on nature as a whole, for example the Australian Great Barrier Reef's annual sex festival, is a time when a huge release of sperm and eggs are released into the ocean. This whole event is triggered by the full moon in November, and takes place every year.[13]

The subconscious mind can be viewed as your inner Garden of Eden, and whatever seeds are nurtured within that garden become your habitual nature. It all depends on what you focus your attention on, ultimately, watering particular seeds while letting others perish. People born under fixed signs (Taurus, Leo, Scorpio and Aquarius) may find it more difficult to change their habits than those of mutable or cardinal signs, in such cases more effort is needed to keep up the momentum and focus on the new goals, as opposed to falling back into old habits.

There is an old analogy, a fight between two wolves which live within you, one is good and the other is bad. A wise old monk was once teaching his student about this concept, he said to the boy:

"A fight is going on inside me, a constant battle between two wolves. One is bad, consumed with greed, anger, bitterness, self-pity, regret, resentment, jealousy, envy, and ego. The other is good, he is full of optimism, peace, hope, humility, empathy, kindness, compassion and love.
The boy asked the monk "Which wolf will win?"
The monk replied, "The one you feed."

Notes for chapter 3

(1) Jimmy Swartz, One meal a day, a history of how eating evolved, The omad diet, April 2018, Omaddiet.com. https://omaddiet.com/1-meal-a-day/

(2) Kris Gunnars BSc, 10 evidence based health benefits of intermittent fasting, Healthline, newsletter, Aug 2016. https://www.healthline.com/nutrition/10-health-benefits-of-intermittent-fasting

(3) Karen Feldscher, In pursuit of healthy aging, health and medicine, The Harvard Gazette. Nov 2017. https://news.harvard.edu/gazette/story/2017/11/intermittent-fasting-may-be-center-of-increasing-lifespan/

(4) NIH / National institute of Aging, Longer daily fasting times improve health and longevity in mice, Science News, Science daily, Sept 2018, https://www.sciencedaily.com/releases/2018/09/180906123305.htm

(5) Jo Willey, Eat less, live longer: Cutting back on food can help repair the body says new study. Express, Health, 2014. https://www.express.co.uk/life-style/health/465647/Eat-less-live-longer-Cutting-back-on-food-can-help-repair-the-body-says-new-study

(6) Dhammagavesi Bhikkhu, How often and how much do buddhist monks eat a day in monasteries?, Meditation centre, Quora. https://www.quora.com/How-often-and-how-much-do-buddhist-monks-eat-a-day-in-monasteries

(7) Fasting, Buddhism, Wikipedia, https://en.wikipedia.org/wiki/Fasting

(8) Sleep habits of lions, National Sleep Foundation,
https://sleep.org/articles/sleep-habits-of-lions/

(9) What's the best time of the day to nap? National Sleep
Foundation,
https://sleep.org/articles/whats-the-best-time-of-the-day-to-
nap/

(10) Rob Stein, Midday naps found to help fend off heart
disease, Washington Post, Feb 2007.
http://www.washingtonpost.com/wp-dyn/content/article/20
07/02/12/AR2007021200626.html?noredirect=on

(11) Claudine Morgan, When`s the best time to workout? July
4th 2016,
http://greatist.com/fitness/whats-best-time-work-out

(12) Lunar Effect, wikipedia,
https://en.wikipedia.org/wiki/Lunar_effect

(13) BEC Crew, The Full Moon Just Triggered One of The
Largest Mass Spawning Events of 2016, Nature, Science alert.
https://www.sciencealert.com/the-full-moon-just-triggered-o
ne-of-the-largest-mass-spawning-events-of-2016

Chapter 4, Nature's bounty

Our perceived reality is the projection of our combined consciousness within the energy fields surrounding us. Food is just another form of energy, vibrating at a given frequency. Nature's bounty is full of fresh, nutritious, quality foods grown within the Sun's life giving properties. These energetic frequencies are transferred to the body on consumption. In contrast corporate foods, highly processed, lacking in life, light and nutrition, give us little of real value. For the mind and body to be in harmony, in good health, and functioning within a balanced consciousness, it needs a moderate supply of fresh vitamins and minerals. A modest supply in modest proportions should be enough to satisfy the mind's desire for more nutrients.

Highly processed corporate foods with cheap ingredients, preservatives and additives contain quantity without quality, consequently, the lack of vital nutrients convince the mind and body that it is still hungry. An unfulfilled diet turns the individual into an enlarged unfulfilled person, an unhappy and ineffective addition to the human collective. With corporate food one will develop a corporate appetite, a corporate body and finally become a corpse.

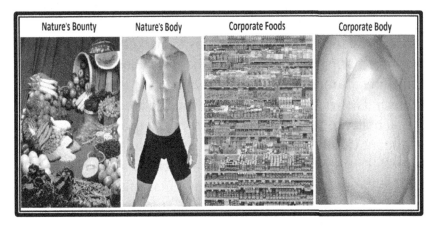

Nature's Bounty   Nature's Body   Corporate Foods   Corporate Body

GMO

Our food is being tampered with, and has been for a long time. Genetically Modified Organisms (GMO) are the result of a laboratory process. Genes from the DNA of one species are extracted and artificially merged with the genes of a different plant or animal. The foreign genes may have originated from bacteria, viruses, insects, animals or even humans. Some of the world's largest global agricultural companies, specialising in GMO seeds, have produced what are called suicide seeds. GURT (Genetic use restriction technology), is a genetic modification which causes the second generation of seeds to be sterile, forcing the grower to turn to the seed producer for their annual supply.

India, one of the world's largest producers of cotton was targeted by one of these huge corporations as part of their conquest for seed control around the globe. From the mid 80's, a company which I shall not name, beginning with M, modified their cotton seeds with a gene which turned them into suicide seeds, allowing them to benefit financially from royalties, claiming they had created something new, where in fact they had just perverted an existing seed found in nature. The intellectual rights relating to seeds, something nature produces for free is widely considered as a fraudulent scam. The globalisation project over the past 20 years has allowed these companies to infiltrate domestic markets all over the world, replacing diversity by overshadowing localised varieties found in nature, natural varieties which have evolved over thousands of years which thrive in specific areas. The one size fits all policy of these GMO seeds, competing against nature's abundant varieties and natural selection is staggeringly naive. With their vast wealth these companies have managed to lock local markets into licensing arrangements, influence local and regional governments, coerce huge swathes of the farming community, and expand their global monopoly. With glossy literature and slick promotional videos, thousands of Indian farmers, of modest means have been lured into the world of M's GMO seeds. They were offered loans only if they would use the new seeds and pesticides, promising better yields. Costing many times more than the local variety, these GMO seeds didn't always perform as expected, throwing many farmers into financial debt, even ruin. Some unable to pay their loans were forced to turn their land and what little assets they had over to these unscrupulous corporations, in the end many farmers took their own lives. Ironically the suicide seeds brought about suicide farmers. 95% of India's cotton seeds are now controlled by M, over the past 20 years over 291,000 Indian farmers have committed suicide under the pressure of crippling debt. M has been heavily criticised and accused of contributing to these appalling statistics. In 2009 alone 17,638 Indian farmers committed suicide, that's 1 every 30 minutes. The other problem associated with GMO crops is cross contamination, gene pollution, or genetic drift. Over time it is inevitable that the GMO crops will encroach and pollute organic farms, turning their natural crops into the intellectual property of the large agricultural corporations who own the GMO technical patents. The Corporations claim they are trying to help feed the world and fight famine in under developed countries. In reality they are expanding their monopolies, gaining more control of the food supply and manipulating the situation to make the world's farmers dependent on their seeds and pesticides.[1][2] The debate over the safety of GMO will go on for decades, the long term effects on human biology is still in its infancy. The introduction of new genes into fruit or vegetables may result in new toxins, new bacteria, new allergens, and even new diseases.[3] What is clear is the increase in global control and dependency of our food supply, once free, is now in the hands of the international corporations. Science is a tool which can be used for good or bad, it is certainly clever but not always wise. In the hands of a psychopathic corporation with a profit centred agenda, the results can be devastating, a negative benefit to the overall good of humanity. The control of the cotton seeds is only the beginning. The objectives of these giant corporations is to do away with natural seed diversity, from which they cannot profit from, substituting all seeds with their artificial patented versions, eventually controlling everything we grow and eat. Genetically modified seeds produce genetically modified foods; genetically modified foods genetically modify those who wish to eat them. The natural balance of frequencies within nature's bounty are being carelessly tampered with, something humanity may never recover from.

Processed foods

The main reason for processing food is to eliminate micro-organisms and extend shelf life. The closer your diet is to nature the better the food is for your body. Each process destroys valuable nutrients and alters some properties. Simply cooking, chopping or combining one food with another is considered a process, and exposing food to high levels of heat, light and/or oxygen will also reduce its nutrient value. Vitamins B and C can be washed out especially during the boiling process. It is preferable to eat vegetables as close to raw as practically possible, keeping intact the delicate vitamins, minerals, photochemical, antioxidants and enzymes. The greater the heat and longer the cooking time the greater the nutrient destruction. When the body craves nutrients, chemicals are produced giving the feeling of hunger, when nutrient rich foods are consumed the body and mind become satisfied, a balanced chemistry will hold off the hunger feeling for a healthy amount of time, keeping the body trim. If the individual consumes dead food, lacking in essential nutrients but full of calories, the body will overeat and still feel hungry, unable to satisfy a craving for nutrients, the body soon expands, blossoming towards obesity. In this modern age of plenty the United States has developed a problem with an overweight population. Submerged in fast corporate living, two out of every three adults are overweight. One third is considered obese.[4] This problem gets worse each year, spreading around the west like a virus, influenced by one another's behavioural patterns. Overweight people are contributing to the human collective with their gluttonous appetite for non nutritious corporate processed foods.

Typical nutrient losses for vitamins and minerals during the cooking process

Nutrient	Freeze	Dry	Cook	Cook+Drain	
Vitamin A	5%	50%	25%	35%	10%
Retinol Activity Equivalent		5%		50%	25%
Alpha Carotene		5%	50%	25%	35%
Beta Carotene	5%	50%	25%	35%	10%
Beta Cryptoxanthin		5%	50%	25%	35%
Lycopene	5%	50%	25%	35%	10%
Lutein+Zeaxanthin		5%	50%	25%	35%
Vitamin C	30%	80%	50%	75%	50%
Thiamin	5%	30%	55%	70%	40%
Riboflavin	0%	10%	25%	45%	5%
Niacin	0%	10%	40%	55%	5%
Vitamin B6	0%	10%	50%	65%	45%
Folate	5%	50%	70%	75%	30%
Food Folate	5%	50%	70%	75%	30%
Folic Acid	5%	50%	70%	75%	30%
Vitamin B12	0%	0%	45%	50%	45%
Calcium	5%	0%	20%	25%	0%
Iron	0%	0%	35%	40%	0%
Magnesium	0%	0%	25%	40%	0%
Phosphorus	0%	0%	25%	35%	0%
Potassium	10%	0%	30%	70%	0%
Sodium	0%	0%	25%	55%	0%
Zinc	0%	0%	25%	25%	0%
Copper	10%	0%	40%	45%	0%

In 2008 a study was conducted and published in the Journal of Agriculture and Food Chemistry. The study concluded that raw broccoli appears to deliver anti-cancer compounds 10 times more efficiently than cooked broccoli.[5] Another study conducted at the Roswell Park Cancer Institute in Buffalo, found that eating small amounts of raw broccoli and cabbage over a period of time, reduced the risk of bladder cancer by as much as 40%.[6] There is little doubt that eating plenty of fresh minimally processed, high quality vegetables, is one of the best ways to stay healthy.

Breakfast cereals

The breakfast cereal found in many family homes has been promoted by big corporations as the natural way to start the day. Many cereals are produced from a process called extrusion where grains are mixed with water to form slurry. This mixture is then forced through an extruder, a tiny hole shaping each cereal at high temperature and pressure. After expanding they are sprayed with a mixture of sugar and oil, an overall process which destroys most of the initial nutrients that the grain once offered. Many studies have been conducted to see what the effects are from living on these cereals for prolonged periods. One such study in 1960 at the University of Michigan, a tongue in cheek study, experimented on three groups of rats. The first group were fed on cornflakes and water. Group two were fed on the cardboard box which the cereal came in and water. The third group were fed on rat chow with water. As expected the third group stayed relatively healthy, the second group, fed on the box, became lethargic, eventually dying of malnutrition. What astounded the research team was the death of the first group eating the cornflakes, they died before the rats that where fed on the box, furthermore before death they threw fits, bit each other and finally died of convulsions. The experiment was not meant to be a serious study but the results were far from funny. It has been suggested that the extrusion process breaks down the organelles and disperse the proteins which then become toxic.[7]

PH of the body

The bodies PH balance is important for maintaining good health. It has been known for decades how detrimental an acidic diet can be to the human body. Unprocessed foods found throughout nature generally lean towards the alkaline side of the PH scale; occasionally we find some natural foods being mildly acidic. Foods full of naturally occurring nutrients promote health and keep the bodies PH in good order. Processed foods on the other hand tend to be more acidic, contributing to an increase in health problems for people throughout developed countries, who find themselves being seduced by advertising and other social pressures, into consuming highly processed acidic foods. Excess acid in the body can lead to many problems such as indigestion, nausea, bloating, gout, cataracts, constipation, strokes, allergies, heart disease, diabetes, osteoporosis and cancer. Research has shown a link between acid PH and cancer. Cancer thrives in an acidic environment, producing lactic acid as it grows. Some research scientists suspect a link between PH, candida and cancer. The yeast fungus called candida is present in all of us, when the fungus overwhelms the gut's probiotic presence the candida becomes an overall health threat. Cancer tumours have been found to reside amongst candida colonies. It appears that the best way to keep the gut healthy and the candida under control is to consume fresh alkaline foods within nature's bounty.[8]

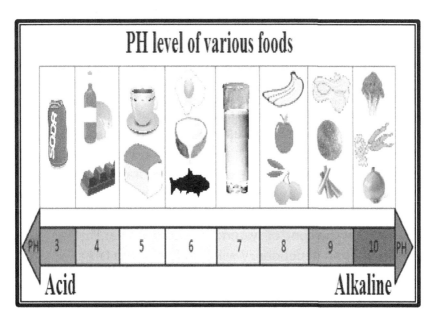

Before the expansion of modern super markets, most foods were bought and produced locally, keeping them fresh and close to nature's source. The average family also grew a limited selection of fruit and vegetables in their own gardens, contributing to a healthier lifestyle. Processed packaged foods are convenient for the modern, time poor, corporate worker, but generally not as good for their health. Pre-made boxed meals, microwaved, ready to eat in 10 minutes is a recipe for disaster. No wonder developed countries are seeing an explosion in the rates of cancer, diabetes and other life threatening illnesses.

They say, you are what you eat, to a certain extent this is true. The human body on one hand is delicate and fragile but on the other hand robust and resilient. What we put into our bodies is far more important than what most people realise. Outside our five senses, within the electrical universe everything is giving off a frequency, food is no exception. Nature provides us with an abundance of perfect foods found throughout the world, helping to sustain a healthy balance of mind and body, keeping communication flowing between all levels of consciousness. These natural foods harness life giving energy emanating from the Sun, which eventually is passed onto us. Highly processed foods lose that energy. In their arrogance the corporations try to compete with this balance, they pervert nature at the DNA level with profit motivated science, trying to control all aspects of our food production, supply and consumption, even to the point of how we cook the food. The main objective of these corporations is to entice you away from healthy self-sufficiency, into a life of unhealthy dependency on their inferior products. Linked at the higher levels within the control system, it becomes clear that processed food dependency will also favour the large pharmaceutical corporations, offering medications and temporary relief for symptoms brought about by poor nutrition. Through long term dependency on drugs and medical procedures, the big pharmaceutical corporations profit from long drawn out treatments to which many people would have been better off using natural remedies, better diet and/or life style changes. The further we drift away from nature the more detrimental it is to our overall health.

In a capitalist style democracy, the relationship between Government policy and the prosperity of commerce and industry are very much interlinked. When I was 11, in 1979, Margaret Thatcher's Tory government came to power in the United Kingdom. At that time school meals had become a long tradition for all British school children. An important contribution towards providing a healthy balanced diet for the masses. Before Thatcher, the school and local authority would carefully design a variety of balanced, well portioned, meals for all children to enjoy. This all changed when nutritional standards were scrapped in favour of competitive tendering. The traditional school meal was contracted out to the private sector, replacing school kitchens with snack bars and canteen styled dining rooms. The old modest portioned, balanced meal was replaced by a selection of fast foods like chips, beans, pies, sausages and burgers.[9] I personally remember the change which took place at my school around 1982. I was so appalled at the choice on offer that i went home for dinner following the changes.

Although most people In western countries contribute to their government's finances, some of these institutions are increasingly coming under pressure to balance the nation's books. With an aging population, they are struggling to cope with the increase in post pension hand outs. Consequently, they needed an alternative option which would give them a way out. They realised, a long time ago, in projected models, that they could not afford to support millions of healthy old people. One way around this was to promote unhealthy eating and drinking habits early on. This had to be done in such a way that it would be seen as a personal free market choice. And the people it was targeted at, who became obese and sick in the process, only had themselves to blame. In the mean time those organisations promoting such policies increased revenue for the government from various sources including fast food giants, pharmaceutical corporations and the medical profession.

Very little happens in this world, especially on the scale of western obesity, that is not planned by government agencies, think tanks or policy makers. It is meant to happen. There are many environmental factors known as 'defaults' which influence people's day to day lives, in subtle yet sophisticated ways. Countries which are suffering from an obesity epidemic have slowly created a set of environmental defaults which are contributing to their population's rise in obesity. In a 2012 summary of a selection of reports produced by the Organisation for Economic Cooperation and Development (OECD) presented in a document entitled 'Role of Policy and Government in Obesity Epidemic' it was stated:

"The OECD supported the idea that regulatory and fiscal policy could reduce obesity by improving defaults for the whole population"- Nicole L. Novak and Kelly D. Brownell[10]

It appears that the recent huge expansion of fast food outlets throughout the private sector, have been allowed, and even encouraged, by city planners and government policy makers, because it suits their overriding agenda. The system of control which works behind the scenes to promote and expand the globalisation project is a well oiled machine which has evolved over a very long time. Your controllers, the established elite, have a sinister plan for the future of humanity, and in order to achieve their goals, the vast majority of their subordinates need to be divided, undermined and dis-empowered, in order to prevent any form of cohesive unions from threatening their hegemony. They are a small club above all elected politicians, bureaucrats and civil servants, with sub-clubs beneath specialising in specific areas of social change. The further the globalisation project advances, the more control, order and restrictions will be placed on humanity, increasing vaccines, pharmaceutical drug consumption, along with more electromagnetic pollution. With a global or international, one size fits all policy, problems produced by those policies will be replicated across the board. Each generation is subjected to more unnatural stimuli than the previous one, pulling them further away from their natural harmonious balance with nature's rhythms and cycles.

"Diet, injections and injunctions will combine, from a very early age, to produce the sort of character and the sort of beliefs that the authorities consider desirable, and any serious criticism of the powers that be will become psychologically impossible." – Bertrand Russel – The Impact of Science on Society

As each new generation is steered towards new socialised norms of political correctness, fitting neatly into the cogs of projected government initiatives and public policy, their basic grounding coordinates of morality in comparison to previous generations become distorted. And as the decades pass, those social norms and moral compasses, which were once took for granted will disappear in a vacuum of stimulated trends, fads and fashions. Consequently, what we consider normal behavior today has been manufactured, the only true lasting foundation of the human conscious relationship with nature, the macrocosm and the Logos is the information contained within the zodiac. Its profound synchronicity and poetical wisdom has stood unchanged for over 5000 years. It is our only true benchmark to nature, our real heritage to ancient history and a guide to the universal parameters of truth. Consequently, astrology has been the target of ridicule by the establishment and mainstream mouthpieces for years, usually by those who know very little about the subject. If you undermine all levels of unity within society, the people will never be able to come together to oppose the system which controls them. The increase in obesity may be another initiative designed to undermine the health of a nation along with a decline in social cohesion. It is therefore up to the individual to take back control of their own eating habits and overall lives, in order to become the best version of themselves in the short time they are here.

Agenda 21 (sustainable development in the 21st century)

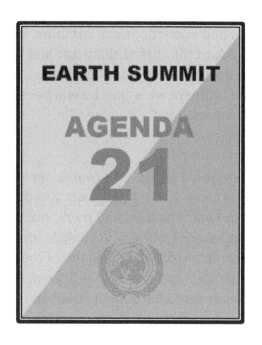

In the summer of 1992, in Rio de Janeiro, Brazil, a United Nations conference was organised, called the Earth Summit, also known as Agenda 21. Its overall objective was to promote sustainable development for the future of mankind and the planet in general for the coming 21st century. By the end of the summit 178 countries had signed up to its proposed initiatives which included the following:[11][12]

- The phasing out of national sovereignty.
- The phasing out of private property.
- State control, planning and management of all land resources.
- Restructuring of the family unit, along with state management and interference of the raising of all children.
- The creation of human settlement zones.
- Job allocation by the state, within the state and for the state.
- Mass migration and resettlement as people are moved away from rural areas into human settlement zones.
- Restructuring of the educational system, to prepare the next generation into accepting Agenda 21.
- Mass global depopulation to a sustainable level.

It appears that in order for the United Nations to achieve its ultimate objectives, the majority of the human race must be domesticated towards their goals, while at the same time undermining any possibility of resistance. Individual rights will need to be curtailed in favour of those who are steering the collective. Although obesity was on a steady increase prior to 1992, the rate of increase seems to have accelerated at an alarming rate after the implementation of Agenda 21.

"The United Nations Decade of Education for Sustainable Development (2005-2014) sought to mobilize the educational resources of the world to help create a more sustainable future. - The overall goal of the UN Decade of Education for Sustainable Development (DESD) was to integrate the principles, values and practices of sustainable development into all aspects of education and learning. This educational effort encouraged changes in behaviour that created a more sustainable future in terms of environmental integrity, economic viability and a just society for present

and future generations." - UN Decade of Education for Sustainable Development, UNESCO.[13]

To distinguish between being overweight or obese a simple body mass index (BMI) calculation is produced, in which a person's weight (kg) is divided by the square of his or her height (m). A person with a BMI equal or over 25 falls in the overweight range, anyone with 30 or above is considered obese.

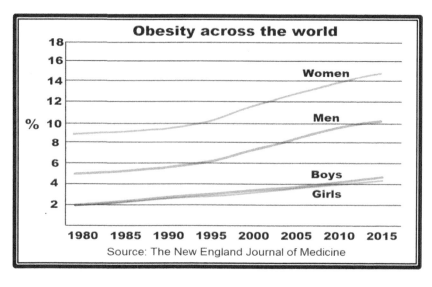

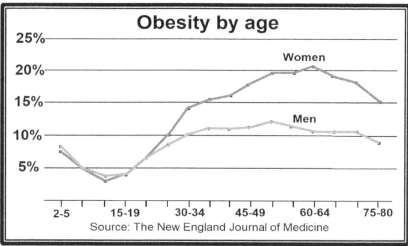

What stands out above all else, from the previous two graphs, is the number of women in comparison to men suffering from obesity. The Sun and Moon have traditionally represented the male and female in both astrology and ancient cultures. Women are considered to be more internal, sensitive and in tune with their emotions, representing all the things associated with the Moon's metaphysical characteristics. Men on the other hand reflect the Sun's characteristics, concerning the focal aspect of consciousness, the ego and all the Sun's attributes concerning the physical realm. This fact that women are more susceptible than men with regard to weight gain may have something to do with the female's traditional metaphysical make up and greater connection to the spiritual subconscious. The metaphysical differences between men and women are explored in greater depth in my 2017 book '*Metaphysics of the Gods*'.

The United States, home of the United Nations, has the worst rates of overweight and obesity out of all the world's developed countries. At present, seven states have a population obesity rate above 35%, with West Virginia leading the field with a staggering 38.1% having a BMI equal or over 30. Although America is one of the last countries to preserve the right to bear arms. A provision placed within the constitution to repel any challenge to their republic, foreign or domestic. The fact that so many Americans are shockingly overweight may eliminate any advantage, rendering them vulnerable to a loss of sovereignty.

Juvenal was a Roman satirical poet (circa 100AD), who came up with the phrase 'bread and circuses'.

"Juvenal who originated the phrase, used it to decry the selfishness of common people and their neglect of wider concerns. The phrase implies a population's erosion or ignorance of civic duty as a priority." - bread and circuses[14]

Depopulation agenda

Together with the desire to eradicate national sovereignty there is a push to depopulate the planet to a manageable level, all part of agenda 21's sustainable development. Many elitists throughout history have desired the culling of those who they consider as 'useless eaters', they are eugenicists. Over the centuries they have callously sent millions of young men to their deaths in unnecessary conflicts against their own relatives in other countries.

"Of all the problems which will have to be faced in the future, in my opinion, the most difficult will be those concerning the treatment of the inferior races of mankind." — Leonard Darwin (son of Charles Darwin)[15]

"I just wonder what it would be like to be reincarnated in an animal whose species had been so reduced in numbers that it was in danger of extinction. What would be its feelings toward the human species whose population explosion had denied it somewhere to exist... I must confess that I am tempted to ask for reincarnation as a particularly deadly virus." - Prince Philip Duke of Edinburgh.[16]

"The world today has 6.8 billion people, that's heading up to about 9 billion. Now if we do a really great job on new vaccines, health care, reproductive health services, we could lower that by perhaps 10 or 15%"- Bill Gates TED conference 2012[17]

In 1979, at about the same time Margaret Thatcher was moving into 10 Downing Street, an unknown organisation erected six giant granite stones in Elbert County, Georgia. The inscriptions on the stones support the idea of sustainable development and depopulation, known as the Georgia Guidestones. The monument conveys a set of 10 guidelines in

8 modern languages and 4 ancient ones. Today's global population is approximately 7.125 billion. The proposal is to reduce this down to a mere 500 million, a staggering 93% reduction.

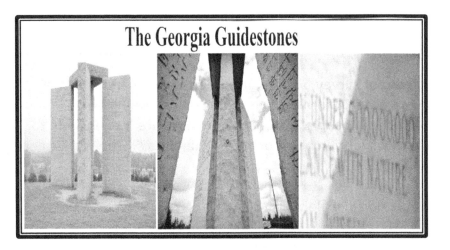

The Georgia Guidestones

There are many ways to promote depopulation without resorting to brutal systemic slaughter of undesirables. More sophisticated, yet subtle, ways of persuasion are used to distract each new generation from participating in population expansion.

Lifestyle choice. Living as a single person is no longer seen as a social stigma.

"In 2017, the U.S. census reported 110.6 million unmarried people over the age of 18—that's 45.2 percent of the American adult population—carrying out their lives to a new set of societal norms." - Observer 2018[18]

The promotion of LGBT lifestyles. No longer regarded as taboo.

"Drawing on the widest survey of sexual behaviour since the Kinsey Report, David Spiegelhalter, in his book Sex By

Numbers, answers key questions about our private lives. Here he reveals how Kinsey's contested claim that 10% of us are gay is actually close to the mark." - The Guardian 2015[19]

Debt has become an acceptable burden to a whole new generation, who consider it as the norm. Putting many people off having a family due to financial worries.

"A recent survey by the National Association of Consumer Bankruptcy Attorneys says members are seeing a big increase in people whose student loans are forcing them to delay major purchases or starting families." - The Wall Street Journal 2012[20]

Reduction in male sperm counts.

"News last week that sperm counts in western men have halved confirmed what experts already knew. The real problem is that no one knows why" - The Guardian 2017[21]

Choosing a career over motherhood.

"According to a recent New York Post article, 43 percent of college-educated women between the ages of 33 and 46 are childfree. And many of these women appear to be bypassing motherhood altogether, as opposed to simply postponing it." - Psychology Today, 2011.[22]

Before the intrusion of large governments, imposing their will in nearly every aspect of our lives, most people were relatively self sufficient, much of their food was produced locally or by themselves in small garden allotments. Their diets were generally healthier and closer to nature. Before big governments, big banks and big wars, the people who lived before the 20th century rarely died from diseases like cancer or diabetes. With the expansion of the industrial revolution and the migration of millions of people from rural communities into the cities, the need for storable foods increased. Food companies sprang up producing products en masse, mixing nature's bounty with artificial chemicals and preservatives which would enhance the taste and give their products a longer shelf life. Unfortunately during these processes the nutritional value of the original foods became distorted, overtaken by the detrimental effects of the chemicals used in the preservation process.

The accumulative effect of chemicals

It is possible that the accumulative effect of synthetic chemical additives found in today's foods could be responsible for a multitude of unwanted side effects. Could this be a leading cause behind today's increase in a wide variety of modern diseases? Some scientists seem to think so.

"Chemicals have replaced bacteria and viruses as the main threat to human health...The diseases we're beginning to see as the major causes of death in the latter part of this century and into the 21st century are diseases of chemical origin." - Rick Irvin Toxicologist Texas A&M University[23]

"There are two big -- and by big I mean monumental -- problems with the argument and the perspective taken by federal regulatory agencies and by the manufacturers of foods and medicines. The argument is that trace levels of these chemicals do no harm to human health. What that argument ignores is the cumulative effect of hundreds, if not thousands, of these chemicals entering and then mixing within the human body. This is known as the "body burden." We each carry a "body burden" of these synthetic chemicals." - Randall Fitzgerald, Author of 'The hundred year lie'[24]

Sugar (shukra)

The word 'sugar' is derived from the word 'shukra', the Sanskrit word for the planet Venus. The link between excessive sugar consumption and weight gain is well documented, its main problem is that it is a major calorie source with little or no nutritional value. The chemical process within the body, which promotes fat storage is relatively straight forward, it basically revolves around insulin levels. When the body is chemically balanced and working normally, food is digested in the gut releasing glucose into the bloodstream, this in turn triggers beta cells within the pancreas to increase the level of insulin which then allows the glucose to be used by the body's cells for energy. The greater the insulin levels the greater the metabolism of glucose. If energy released from this glucose is not used during our daily energy expenditure it eventually becomes stored in the body's cells as fat deposits. When all our food is digested and glucose levels in the blood subside, insulin levels reduce accordingly. This changes the body's metabolism over from fat storage to fat usage, and all those little fat deposits stored within the body's cells start to break down into usable forms of energy. Consequently, the longer the fasting process between meals, the longer the fat burn period, brought about by low levels of insulin.

Studies relating to insulin and weight gain

In a recent study reported by the Intensive dietary management website, 14 diabetics were given oral insulin over a six month period. Their insulin levels were steadily increased up to 100 units per day. By the end of the study their body weight had increased on average by 19lbs, furthermore, this was in spite of a reduction in daily food consumption, by an average 300 calories each. Although the patients ate less they put on a significant amount of weight, suggesting it was the insulin not the calories driving weight gain.

"What happens when we give high doses of insulin to patients? Insulin makes you gain weight. The more insulin you take, the more weight you gain. It almost doesn't matter how much you eat or how much you try to exercise. The weight just keeps coming on." - IDM (Intensive dietary management), insulin causes weight gain.[25]

In another study conducted with 708 diabetics, oral insulin was added to their treatment. As expected they gained weight. The patients who received the highest doses of insulin gained the most while those on the low doses gained the least.

"Under the influence of insulin, our body receives instructions to "gain fat". In response, we eat more and/or decrease energy expenditure. It is not a voluntary act. - The question is NOT how to balance calories, the question is how to balance our hormones. In most cases, the crucial question is not how to reduce calories but how to reduce insulin." - IDM (Intensive dietary management), insulin causes weight gain.[25]

"UT Southwestern Medical Center researchers have identified a crucial link between high levels of insulin and pathways that lead to obesity." - UT Southwestern Medical Center[26]

Insulin resistance

This is a condition where the body's cells fail to respond normally to varying levels of insulin, consequently, as glucose enters the blood more insulin is produced to counteract the body's resistance, promoting weight gain, as more insulin means more fat storage. If insulin resistance is not reversed it can lead to type 2 diabetes along with an increased risk of weight gain. The condition is promoted by a habitual high intake of too much sugar, fructose and carbohydrates, at regular intervals, interfering with the body's natural ability to reset its overall chemical balance. To reverse the detrimental slide towards insulin resistance a low sugar/carbohydrate diet needs to be implemented along with periods of fasting. The abuse of alcohol, through binge drinking, will also contribute to insulin resistance.

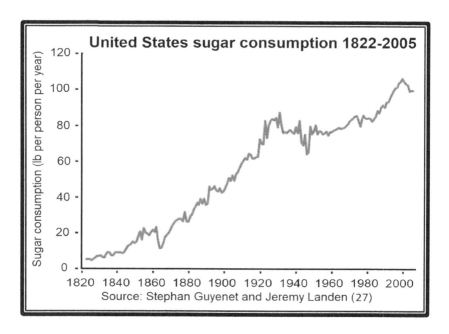

Western society is consuming far too much sugar. (WHO) the World Health Organization have recently reduced their recommendation for a person's sugar consumption down to no more than 5% of their total energy intake, this is equivalent to approximately 25 grams or 6 teaspoons per day.[28] However, the average American today consumes 19.5 teaspoons per day or 82 grams.[29] When taking into account that a small 12 oz can of coke contains an alarming 39 grams of sugar, anyone who consumes a modest soft drink smashes their daily sugar allowance in minutes.[30]

Insulin sensitivity

By eating a high sugar/carbohydrate diet at regular intervals the body loses its sensitivity towards insulin, this is comparable to the drug addict needing larger amounts of the drug to achieve the same result. The body is the same with insulin, abusing it with a constant stream of sugar/carb will reduce its sensitivity. It is thought that around 1/3 of the worlds population has some degree of insulin resistance, promoting greater levels of insulin which turns off the fat burn process. What they need is the opposite, insulin sensitivity. When the body is sensitive to insulin less of the hormone needs to be produced to achieve the desired effect reducing the chance of weight gain. To reverse an insulin resistant metabolism, changes need to be made, to give your body a break from the unhealthy onslaught of high sugar/carb consumption. According to Thomas Delauer, a fitness and optimisation coach, implementing a sugar/carbs starvation diet for 2-3 days, together with intermittent fasting, can help reset the body's sensitivity to insulin.[31] Low insulin levels also trigger the body's natural healing process to take place, restoring balance and overall health. There are a variety of great foods which will promote insulin sensitivity, foods low in sugars and carbohydrates. More exercise and more sleep will also improve insulin sensitivity.

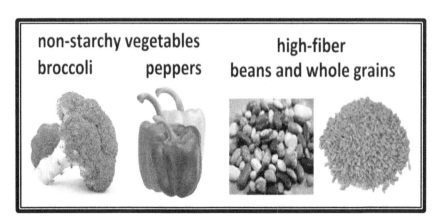

non-starchy vegetables
broccoli   peppers

high-fiber
beans and whole grains

protein-rich
meats, fish, nuts

antioxidant
berries

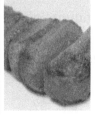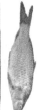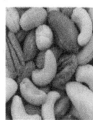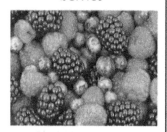

lower GI sweet potatoes   unsweetened teas

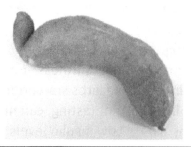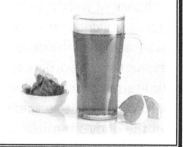

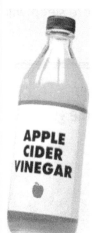

Apple Cider Vinegar

1) Antibacterial properties
2) Contains beneficial minerals,
   (potassium, magnesium, iron and calcium)
3) Lowers blood sugar levels
4) Increases insulin sensitivity
5) Helps reduce weight
6) Helps lower cholesterol
7) Improves digestion

Add 2 tablespoons to a glass of water with a slice of lemon.

Testimonies concerning fasting and health improvements

The concept of fasting to reset the bodies chemical equilibrium, in order to promote its natural healing potential, has been known about for thousands of years. Various studies have been conducted to determine the positive effects fasting can have regarding ill health.

Testimonial (1)
Asthma, bronchitis, sinusitis, eczema

"After I had asthma attacks that led to a serious case of bronchitis, I decided to register at the Hawaii Naturopathic Retreat Center to undergo a supervised water fast. I had chronic sinusitis for many years that required me to always keep with me something with which I could blow my nose. I also had chronic eczema, which was especially bad on my heels. That night, as I began my fast, I had a typical asthma attack, but took no medications to quell it. It took more than two hours before I could breath well enough to go back to sleep. That is the last time that I had such an attack. My water fast lasted 14 days, most of which were spent resting at the center, as my energy levels were expectedly low. Rest was what I needed, so no conflict there. Like the asthma symptoms, the sinus congestion also disappeared, and the crusty, cracking eczema on my heels gradually improved 95% so that they are now close to normal." - Kurt Lloyd, 49 years old, June 2008.[32]

Testimonial (2)
Chronic back pain, overweight, low energy

"I was feeling like a low energy slug, overweight and burdened with chronic back pain. I spent thousands of dollars on treatments and supplements which gave me partial and temporary relief over years of effort. I fasted for ten days with Maya's guidance, wisdom and care. My pain steadily decreased. I broke my fast on fresh juices and raw organic living foods. Both juices and raw foods are still the main stream of my diet and I love it! I feel so good that I have become a true believer in the power of living nutrition. My tastes have adjusted to enjoy raw simple foods more than other junk. I have more energy and enthusiasm for exercise and have kept my weight off. I am now ten pounds lighter, pain free, happier in my body and brimming with vitality." - Ari Vandershoot, November 2003.[33]

Testimonial (3)
Cyst in ovaries

"Had a 7-9cm cyst in my ovaries that went completely away after three cycles of long fasts. A friend had to get a cyst of a similar size removed with surgery and told me how traumatic it was for her body, so I fasted instead hoping it would help and it did. First was 14 days and I also got my period for the first time in about seven or eight months during that fast. The second, about two or three months after, was three and a half weeks. Then about a month after that i fasted for another week. I had only weak tea and water in the first one, coffee tea and water in the second and third. Was good and really damn easy actually. It also helped with fixing some of my life long food issues, which was the best silver lining to all of this." - Overout Jan 2018.[34]

"According to research conducted by neuroscientist Mark Mattson (Johns Hopkins School of Medicine) and others, cutting your energy intake by fasting several days a week might help your brain ward off neurodegenerative diseases like Alzheimer's and Parkinson's while at the same time improving memory and mood." - Johns Hopkins Health Review.[35]

"Then Jesus was led by the Spirit into the wilderness to be tempted by the devil. After fasting forty days and forty nights, he was hungry. The tempter came to him and said, If you are the Son of God, tell these stones to become bread." - Matthew 4 : 1-3 (NIV)

"While they were worshiping the Lord and fasting, the Holy Spirit said, "Set apart for me Barnabas and Saul for the work to which I have called them." So after they had fasted and prayed, they placed their hands on them and sent them off." - Acts 13 : 2-3 (NIV)

"And one of the multitude answered and said, Master, I have brought unto thee my son, which hath a dumb spirit; And wheresoever he taketh him, he teareth him: and he foameth, and gnasheth with his teeth, and pineth away: and I spake to thy disciples that they should cast him out; and they could not. He answereth him, and saith, O faithless generation, how long shall I be with you? how long shall I suffer you? bring him unto me. And they brought him unto him: and when he saw him, straightway the spirit tare him; and he fell on the ground, and wallowed foaming. And he asked his father, How long is it ago since this came unto him? And he said, Of a child. And ofttimes it hath cast him into the fire, and into the waters, to destroy him: but if thou canst do any thing, have compassion on us, and help us. Jesus said unto him, If thou canst believe, all things are possible to him that believeth. And straightway the father of the child cried out, and said with tears, Lord, I believe; help thou mine unbelief. When Jesus saw that the people came running together, he rebuked the foul spirit, saying unto him, Thou dumb and deaf spirit, I charge thee, come out of him, and enter no more into him. And the spirit cried, and rent him sore, and came out of him: and he was as one dead; insomuch that many said, He is dead. But Jesus took him by the hand, and lifted him up; and he arose. And when he was come into the house, his disciples asked him privately, Why could not we cast him out? And he said unto them, This kind can come forth by nothing, but by prayer and fasting." - Mark 9 : 17-29 (KJV)

"I ate no choice food; no meat or wine touched my lips; and I used no lotions at all until the three weeks were over." - Daniel 10-3 (NIV)

"I fast twice a week and give a tenth of all I get." - Luke 18 : 12 (NIV)

What the Quran says about fasting[36]

"O you who have believed, decreed upon you is fasting as it was decreed upon those before you that you may become righteous." - Quran [2:183]

"[Fasting for] a limited number of days. So whoever among you is ill or on a journey [during them] - then an equal number of days [are to be made up]. And upon those who are able [to fast, but with hardship] - a ransom [as substitute] of feeding a poor person [each day]. And whoever volunteers excess - it is better for him. But to fast is best for you, if you only knew." - Quran [2:184]

"The month of Ramadhan [is that] in which was revealed the Qur'an, a guidance for the people and clear proofs of guidance and criterion. So whoever sights [the new moon of] the month, let him fast it; and whoever is ill or on a journey - then an equal number of other days. Allah intends for you ease and does not intend for you hardship and [wants] for you to complete the period and to glorify Allah for that [to]

which He has guided you; and perhaps you will be grateful." - Quran [2:185]

Low fat / high sugar

Many people fail to appreciate the significance sugar plays in their diet, focusing all their attention on the fat content. As a result, their shopping trolleys are full of low fat foods which contain high levels of sugar. This is a recipe for disaster, and they wonder why they are still putting on weight. Below are a few common foods which contain surprisingly high levels of sugar.

- Yoghurt: Some fat free brands contain high levels of sugar as a counter measure to improve texture and taste after the fat has been removed. A modest serving of 150 grams can contain as much as 20 grams of sugar, nearly all the daily recommended allowance.[37]

- Coleslaw: Made up of shredded vegetables mixed with mayonnaise. Considered a healthy option for many consumers, but within the mayonnaise their is a certain amount of sugar. Each spoonful serving of coleslaw contains on average 1 teaspoon or 4 grams of sugar.[37]

- Bread: Many bread manufacturers add sugar to their mix to enhance the taste, especially highly processed varieties. Some slices can contain as much as 3 grams, almost 1 teaspoon of sugar.[37]

- Fruit Juices: Many supermarket brands of fruit juice contains large amounts of sugar. Some versions contain as much sugar as soft drinks.[38]

- Sports drinks: These drinks have become popular over the past few years, giving people the impression they are the healthy option. However, a standard 570ml bottle contains, on average, 32 grams of added sugar.[38]

- Breakfast cereal: Some cereals contain high levels of added sugar, especially certain varieties aimed at young children. Some have been found to contain as much as 12 grams per 30 gram serving.[38]

Social pressure within the collective

If you are the type of person who is heavily influenced by the people around you, social pressures, fads and fashions, you are more likely to put on weight if you surround yourself with obese people. They say you become like the people you associate with. One reason for this is because a new benchmark of normality develops within the parameters of your view of acceptable behaviour. Within that collective bad eating habits will be generously catered for in a free market environment. It takes a uniquely disciplined individual not to be influenced to some degree by their social collective. A person living in a small town in South East Asia, surrounded by relatively slim people, will develop natural expectations to conform to their social norms within that collective, which will eventually impact their subconscious, sowing new seeds which will change their habitual nature to conform. When a child is brought up by obese parents, the child's fragile, sponge like brain will absorb the behavioral patterns of the parents during those formative years, essentially being programmed by the parent's unhealthy habits. The elephant Ganesha within the child's subconscious is given his coordinates and direction from its early influences. The child will follow in its parent's footsteps, repeating a life of obesity and possible ill health.

Many children, at an early age, are encouraged by their peers to associate brightly coloured, sugar laden beverages with a reward for good behavior or an association with positive emotions. The sweet taste and bright colours will germinate deep rooted seeds within their subconscious which will continue to stimulate urges for the drinks well into the future. Considering the amount of sugar in such drinks and the likelihood of developing insulin resistance through regular consumption, the whole act of introducing children to these drinks is a form of child abuse. Unfortunately most parents are unaware of the associated dangers.

Alcohol (the big bad wolf)

Alcohol and drugs are the domain of the planet Neptune (dreams and illusions). Alcohol is used as a tool to manipulate and seduce people into lowering their bodies resonant vibration. Consequently, it is often referred to as a spirit, this is no accident. After the small window of euphoria has ended, the remaining and lasting effects of consuming alcohol are that of a depressant, pulling those who use it down towards the vibratory frequencies of the base chakra, ruled by Saturn.

The word alcohol is thought to have its origins in the Arabic word 'Al-Khul' or 'Al-Kohl'. Kohl was used in ancient Egypt as an antiseptic, cosmetic and eyeliner. However, it is also thought that 'Al-khul' is the origin for our word ghoul, a reference to a body eating spirit.

"By consuming alcohol into the body, it in effect extracts the very essence of the soul, allowing the body to be more susceptible to neighboring entities most of which are of low frequencies." - Jason Christoff[39]

It is widely promoted in most developed countries as part of an overall strategy to neutralise and destabilise many peoples ability to benefit from their natural balanced equilibrium between their soul (focal mind) and their spirit (subconscious mind). Alcohol will also undermine a person's will power, especially concerning eating habits and life style choices. Once under the influence, those strict guidelines which were leading them towards health, wealth and happiness, can easily go astray, being cast aside for old habits of junk food, binge drinking and tobacco smoking.

Apart from increasing the risk of insulin resistance, the regular use and accumulative effects of alcohol on the body can lead to some serious problems:[40]

- Brain: Alcohol disrupts the brain's communication pathways, affecting behaviour, moods and clarity of thinking.

- Heart: The accumulative effect of too much alcohol, together with binge drinking can damage the heart in a variety of ways. It can cause stretching of the heart muscle, irregular heart beats, together with high blood pressure and the increase risk of a stroke.

- Liver: Although the liver has the ability to regenerate, a constant barrage of alcohol abuse can cause serious damage, with conditions like alcohol induced hepatitis, fatty liver, fibrosis and cirrhosis.

- Pancreas: Alcohol abuse can disrupt the normal functions of the pancreas, leading to poor digestion along with many other complications.

- Cancer: Because alcohol travels all over the body, excessive abuse can promote a variety of cancers. Common ones from drinking are Heart and neck cancer, esophageal cancer, liver cancer, breast cancer and colorectal cancer.

Alcohol abuse can also lower a persons immune system, leaving them vulnerable to diseases like pneumonia and tuberculosis. With all this taken into account, it is understandable that the consumption of alcohol is banned in many countries, cultures and religions. It really is the slow poisoning of the body, and should be avoided if one wishes to be the greatest version of themselves. Consequently, it is important to refrain from drinking any alcohol for at least one full day prior to the new moon, because the body needs to be in its best condition for the fasting and meditation process to achieve the required results.

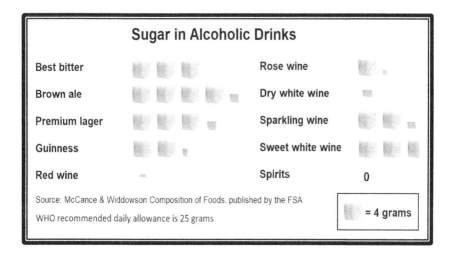

Sugar in Alcoholic Drinks

Best bitter		Rose wine
Brown ale		Dry white wine
Premium lager		Sparkling wine
Guinness		Sweet white wine
Red wine		Spirits 0

Source: McCance & Widdowson Composition of Foods, published by the FSA

WHO recommended daily allowance is 25 grams

= 4 grams

Snacking

If you are determined to snack in the evening, it is vitally important that you choose foods which will not increase your blood sugar, raising a spike in insulin levels. This will break the fasting process and place your body once more in the fat storing mode. It is therefore important to choose your snacks wisely, by opting for something with a low glycemic value (GL). This value is a measure or percentage of glucose in the food, 100 being pure glucose. The secret to avoiding weight gain is basically about what you eat and when you eat it.

Glycemic Index

High GL 70>, Medium GL 56-69, Low GL <55

Grains		Vegetables		Starches		Dairy	
Wheat tortilla	30	Kale	5	Sweet potatoes	48	Butter	0
Wheat pasta	32	Brussels sprouts	6	Brown rice	50	Cheese	0
White pasta	42	Spinach	6	Basmati rice	58	Plain yoghurt	14
Wheat bread	60	Broccoli	10	Couscous	61	Soy milk	30
White bread	70	Cabbage	10	Potatoes	73-78	Milk	31
White Baguette	95	Cauliflower	12	White rice	85	Ice cream	61
		Tomato	15			Rice milk	86

Fruit		Carrots	47	Snacks			
Cherries	22	Green peas	48	Sunflower seeds	18	Drinks	
Grapefruit	25	Corn on the cob	54	Sponge cake	46	Red wine	15
Raspberries	30			Potato crisps	56	Beer	15
Apples	38	Proteins		Blueberry muffin	59	Tomato juice	38
Blueberries	40	Peanuts	21	Raisins	64	Apple juice	44
Strawberries	42	Dried beans	40	Popcorn	65	Orange juice	50
Oranges	46	Lentils	41	Pancake	67	Coca cola	63
Grapes	52	Kidney beans	41	Donuts	76	Sweet soda drinks	68-78
Banana	56	Split peas	45	Porridge oats	79		
Pineapple	59	Chick peas	55	Cornflakes	80	**Source :** (41) (42)	
Watermelon	72	Black eyed beans	59	Rice-cakes	84		

Getting back to nature

"We are star dust we are golden, and we got to get ourselves back to the garden" - Woodstock, Joni Mitchell, 1970.

There is a way out of being trapped in a perpetual unhealthy loop of weight gain, diets and laziness. The first thing to do is to accept there is a problem. Once you admit to yourself that you really have lost control of your dietary habits, only then can you move forward in the right direction. Your new priority is to get back to nature's bounty, along with its timeless rhythms and cycles. Those old habits need to be broken, and there is no time like the present to begin. Consider moving towards the metaphysical diet, introducing periodic moon phase fasting which will help to break old cycles and grow new healthy seeds with positive intent.

There is a system of agriculture known as permaculture (permanent agriculture). A sustainable system based on modest agricultural ecosystems and nature's rhythms and cycles. This concept allows an individual or family to produce most of their own food within a relatively small area which is mostly self regulating and low maintenance.[43] By growing as much of your own food as is practicably possible, you reduce the risk of adverse reactions from the accumulation of synthetic chemicals.

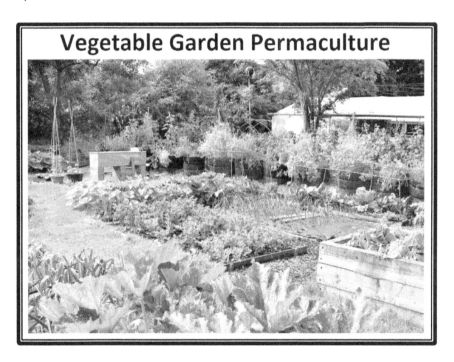

Vegetable Garden Permaculture

Notes for chapter 4

(1) The Seeds Of Suicide: How Monsanto Destroys Farming, Globalresearch.org, http://www.globalresearch.ca/the-seeds-of-suicide-how-monsanto-destroys-farming/5329947

(2) Rising suicide rate for Indian farmers blamed on GMO seeds, RT, November 22, 2014, http://rt.com/news/206787-monsanto-india-farmers-suicides/

(3) BAD SEED: Danger of Genetically Modified Food, https://www.youtube.com/watch?v=go_29vbOdlI

(4) Weight-control Information Network, statistics, website, http://win.niddk.nih.gov/index.htm

(5) Raw broccoli appears to deliver anti-cancer compound 10 times as efficiently as cooked, Journal of Agricultural and Food Chemistry, Oct 25, 2008, http://www.prohealth.com/library/showarticle.cfm?libid=14055

(6) Mike Adams, Natural news, Raw Broccoli, Cabbage Slash Bladder Cancer Risk, http://www.naturalnews.com/023655_Isothiocyanates_raw_foods.html

(7) Dirty Secrets of the Food Processing Industry, The weston a price foundation, http://www.westonaprice.org/health-topics/dirty-secrets-of-the-food-processing-industry/

(8) PF louis, Four things you need to know about cancer and candida, Natural News, December 8th 2012,

http://www.naturalnews.com/038266_cancer_Candida_corre
lations.html
http://www.canceractive.com/cancer-active-page-link.aspx?n
=1089

(9) Rob Lyon's, School dinners: serving up a food sermon,
British school meals have become a tool for social engineering,
Nov 2013.
https://www.spiked-online.com/2013/11/05/school-dinners-s
erving-up-a-food-sermon/

(10) Nicole L. Novak and Kelly D. Brownell, Role of Policy and
Government in the Obesity Epidemic, Circulation Nov 2012,
AHA Journals.org.
https://www.ahajournals.org/doi/abs/10.1161/circulationaha.
111.037929

(11) Agenda 21, wikipedia,
https://en.wikipedia.org/wiki/Agenda_21

(12) Agenda 21 for dummies, Youtube video, Liberalbias100,
2009, https://www.youtube.com/watch?v=TzEEgtOFFlM

(13) UN Decade of Education for Sustainable Development,
UNESCO.
https://en.unesco.org/themes/education-sustainable-develop
ment/what-is-esd/un-decade-of-esd

(14) Bread and circuses, Wikipedia,
https://en.wikipedia.org/wiki/Bread_and_circuses

(15) Leonard Darwin, Quote, good reads,
https://www.goodreads.com/author/quotes/2036161.Leonar
d_Darwin

(16) Prince Philip. Foreword to 'If I Were an Animal' (1987) by Fleur Cowles and Prince Philip.
https://www.amazon.com/If-were-animal-Fleur-Cowles/dp/0688061508

(17) Bill Gates, TED Conference 2012, Presentation, Youtube.
https://www.ted.com/talks/bill_gates?language=en#t-271029

(18) Francesca Friday, More Americans Are Single Than Ever Before—And They're Healthier, Too. Observer, 2018,
https://observer.com/2018/01/more-americans-are-single-than-ever-before-and-theyre-healthier-too/

(19) David Spiegelhalter, Is 10% of the population really gay?. The Guardian 2015.
https://www.theguardian.com/society/2015/apr/05/10-per-cent-population-gay-alfred-kinsey-statistics

(20) Sue Shellenbarger, To Pay Off Loans, Grads Put Off Marriage, Children. The Wall Street Journal, 2012.
https://www.wsj.com/articles/SB10001424052702304818404577350030559887086

(21) Robin Mckie, The infertility crisis is beyond doubt. Now scientists must find the cause. The Guardian, 2017.
https://www.theguardian.com/science/2017/jul/29/infertility-crisis-sperm-counts-halved

(22) Ellen Walker Ph.D. More Women Are Choosing Career over Motherhood: What's Leading This Trend?. Psychology Today, 2011.
https://www.psychologytoday.com/us/blog/complete-without-kids/201108/more-women-are-choosing-career-over-motherhood-what-s-leading

(23) Rick Irvin, toxicologist at Texas A&M University, qtd. in The Hundred-Year Lie by Randall Fitzgerald, pg. 33. https://www.amazon.com/Hundred-Year-Lie-Yourself-Chemic als-Destroying/dp/0452288398

(24) Mike Adams interview with Randall Fitzgerald. Interview with Randall Fitzgerald, author of The Hundred-Year Lie, on the prevalence of toxic chemicals. Natural News, June 2006. https://www.naturalnews.com/019434_harmful_chemicals_p olluted_environment.html

(25) IDM (Intensive dietary management), insulin causes weight gain, hormonal obesity IV. https://idmprogram.com/insulin-causes-weight-gain-hormona l-obesity-iv/

(26) High insulin levels tied to obesity pathways, UT Southwestern Medical Center, Science Daily, 2014. https://www.sciencedaily.com/releases/2014/08/1408251853 19.htm

(27) Stephan Gayenet and Jeremy Landen, Sugar consumption in the US diet between 1822-2005. http://onlinestatbook.com/2/case_studies/sugar.html

(28) WHO, WHO calls on countries to reduce sugars intake among adults and children, http://www.who.int/mediacentre/news/releases/2015/sugar-guideline/en/

(29) UCSF, University of California, How much is too much, Sugar science. http://sugarscience.ucsf.edu/the-growing-concern-of-overcon sumption.html#.W7oBs1QzZdg

(30) Melodie Anne, How many teaspoons of sugar are there in a can of coke, Livingstrong.com. 2017, https://www.livestrong.com/article/283136-how-many-teaspoons-of-sugar-are-there-in-a-can-of-coke/

(31) Thomas Delauer, Training While Fasting: How to Avoid Insulin Resistance, Youtube video, Sept 2017, https://www.youtube.com/watch?v=QfrwYsrqo8I

(32) Kurt Lloyd, 49 years old, June 2008, Fasting testimonials, Hawaii Natuthic Retreat. http://www.hawaiinaturopathicretreat.com/testimonials/fasting-testimonials/

(33) Ari Vandershoot, November 2003, Fasting testimonials, Hawaii Natuthic Retreat. http://www.hawaiinaturopathicretreat.com/testimonials/fasting-testimonials/

(34) Overout, Fasting cured my? What are your stories?, Discussion Post by u/scralchprods. Jan 2018, Reddit. https://www.reddit.com/r/fasting/comments/7mkfkv/fasting_cured_my_what_are_your_stories/

(35) Joe Sugarman, Are there any proven benefits to fasting, Johns Hopkins Health Review, 2016. https://www.johnshopkinshealthreview.com/issues/spring-summer-2016/articles/are-there-any-proven-benefits-to-fasting

(36) Quran verses about Ramadan and fasting. ISLAM.RU. http://islam.ru/en/content/story/quran-verses-about-ramadan-and-fasting

(37) Sugar: Five foods surprisingly high in sugar. Magazine Monitor, BBC News, 2014.

https://www.bbc.com/news/blogs-magazine-monitor-256665
56

(38) Helen West, 18 foods and drinks that are surprisingly high in sugar, Healthline, nutrition, 2016.
https://www.healthline.com/nutrition/18-surprising-foods-high-in-sugar#section6

(39) Jason Christoff, Alcohol and spiritual possession, Christoff Health, 2017.
https://www.jchristoff.com/alcohol-and-spiritual-possession/

(40) NIH (National Institute on Alcohol Abuse and Alcoholism), Alcohol's effect on the body,
https://www.niaaa.nih.gov/alcohol-health/alcohols-effects-body

(41) Valerie Currie, Overview of the glycemic index,
http://valeriecurrie.com/glycemic-index/

(42) Healthjade, What is glycemic (GI) index?
https://healthjade.com/what-is-glycaemic-gi-index/

(43) Permaculture, Wikipedia,
https://en.wikipedia.org/wiki/Permaculture

Chapter 5, Positive mind healing.

As previously mentioned meditation and prayer work together as a mechanism to influence and alter our state and direction of mind, which in turn influences perception of physical reality. The habitual nature of the mind, through the subconscious, can be altered towards a balanced harmonious position, which will effect behaviour. The state of the focal and subconscious mind acts as a spotlight on specific frequencies it is aligned to. Consequently, anger begets more anger and love begets more love, it is the universal law of attraction. The familiarity of a thought will make it much easier to notice and materialise on the outside.

"With our thoughts we make the world." - Gautama Buddha

Metaphysical Healing

The whole idea behind metaphysical healing comes from a holistic approach to illness, where the state of the minds thought processes play a major role in creating either harmony and well-being or disharmony and dis-ease. It is well accepted that a patient stands a far greater chance of recovery if their mental approach to their predicament is a positive one. It is also well documented that depressed people suffer from illness more often than their happier counterparts.[1]

After one understands the mechanisms in place regarding the focal and sub conscious, it becomes clear that anyone with harmonious, balanced awareness is going to have the edge over those individuals who are in a state of perpetual inner conflict. Those at peace riding on the back of the elephant have less chance of becoming physically ill than those who are spilling all their energy fighting both the elephant and the forest.

Everything has a natural sympathetic vibration, a frequency at which it exists in balance and harmony. Even the human body; organs and constituent parts have signature vibrations, a spectrum of frequencies all vibrating in harmony with one another, to reflect the overall health, state of mind and well being of that individual. When various parts of the body fall away from their natural vibratory range, disharmony and dis-ease can manifest.

When two separate systems, vibrating at different frequencies, begin to influence each other, they line up, in order to harmonise. The whole idea behind frequency healing is to ensure the body and its constituent parts vibrate at their natural preferred frequency. When these frequencies drop the immune system suffers, bringing forth illness and dis-ease. Simply by introducing frequency healing tools you can help stimulate the restoration of higher vibrations promoting good health. It has also been found that negative thoughts lower a measured frequency by as much as 12 MHz, whereas positive thoughts do the opposite. Meditation is also beneficial, being one of the best natural contributors in stimulating higher vibrations, by up to 15 MHz.[2]

A great deal of work, on this subject, was conducted back in the 1920s and 30s, by a doctor in America called Royal Raymond Rife MD. He had developed a frequency generator that was purported to cure various diseases, even cancer. This caused a great deal of controversy at the time due to its implications concerning the threat to the established medical profession. It has been suggested that due to its success, at low cost, it was too much of a threat to potential profits of the big pharmaceutical corporations, which was one of the reasons why it was undermined.[3]

"If you want to find the secrets of the universe, think in terms of energy, frequency and vibration." - Nikola Tesla

"We all have the ability to heal ourselves; I know, I have done so... In the morning, know that you are Loved, You Are Love and You Love" - Lisa Bellini

"The words we choose to use when we communicate with each other, carry vibrations. The word 'war' carries a whole different vibration than the word 'peace'. The words we use are showing how we think and how we feel. The careful selection of words, helps to elevate our consciousness and resonate in higher frequencies." - Grigoris Deoudis

"Enlightenment isn't about reaching a destination of "knowing", it is about developing consistent vibrational harmony within one's self and with the surrounding world." - Alaric Hutchinson

"When you continuously give attention to a positive thought, it becomes a dominant thought. Repeating this thought will become a bigger part of your vibration." - Hina Hashmi

Placebo and nocebo

A placebo is either an inert (chemically inactive) substance, or a sham act of surgery, used in drug research trials as a method of producing a control against the genuine act or article. Patients in the trials do not know whether they are on the genuine drug or the placebo. Consequently, those on the placebo are deceived into thinking they are on the genuine treatment, which sometimes produces astonishing results.

"A promising new drug for depression failed to clear efficacy tests this year, illuminating a decades-old problem in psychopharmacology that researchers say deserves more study: the placebo effect, in which patients receiving a dummy pill do almost as well as those on the drug being

tested, thereby wiping out the rationale for the new drug."-
M Enserink, Sciencemag.org[4]

"I've seen people who have had terrible arthritic pain for five or 10 years, receive a placebo injection, stand up, and walk straight out," - Professor Damien Finniss, medical doctor and Associate Professor at the University of Sydney's Pain Management and Research Institute.[5]

During the late 90s a study was carried out on patients with debilitating knee pain. The patients were divided up into three separate groups.

- Group 1) They would have surgery to shave the damaged cartilage in the knee.

- Group 2) They would also have surgery with the joint being flushed out and cleaned.

- Group 3) The placebo group were tricked into believing they had surgery. After sedation an incision was made to the knee then stitched back up.

All three groups went through rehabilitation programs as normal. The results concluded that the placebo group improved just as much as the other two groups who had been through real surgery. They also stated in the conclusion that healthcare researchers should not underestimate the placebo effect regardless of its mechanism.[6]

The placebo is not fully understood, but the simple act of going into a hospital, surrounded by doctors in white coats together with the whole complex of the medical profession, has the ability to trigger deep rooted beliefs within the subconscious, which can influence the patient's outcome whether the real treatment is administered or a placebo.

The beliefs most of us grow up with concerning hospitals and men in white coats comes from years of positive programming by television programs and the media as a whole. Consequently, the nocebo effect can also have unwanted side effects especially if it is administered in the right environment. The nocebo effect occurs when a patient has negative expectations regarding impending treatment. Although an inert substance is administered the patient believes it will have adverse consequences, often, because of the way their subconscious views the medical profession and the doctors, their belief alone will bring on negative symptoms.

Think yourself slim

Being the greatest version of yourself begins with the correct mindset, the right attitude towards yourself, others and the world around you. To develop the right frame of mind for a slim approach to life, many old habits need to be dug up and thrown out. As mentioned previously, the subconscious is like a garden. It can be viewed as your inner Garden of Eden, where seeds germinate into your habitual behaviour. Many seeds were planted before you had a chance to challenge them with a mature focal awareness. Now after years of growth, some seeds have developed very deep roots.

Food has become a curse to some people, with every waking hour drawn to thoughts of eating. Their monkey mind no longer deviates from one subject to the next, it is only interested in the next meal. Three meals a day, at least, with added snacks. They not only feed their enormous stomachs but also all those unhealthy mind weeds which are slowly choking their chances of health, wealth and happiness.

Most people's eating practices happen with little focal attention, choosing the easy option over a healthier choice. When it comes to buying groceries, to many, it is an automatic response to a weekly routine or the occasional bout of hunger. Many people's food shopping expeditions take on the appearance of marauding zombies, with little or no cognitive interaction, they fill their shopping trolleys with the same items week in and week out, most of which has contributed to their weight problem.

In order for new changes to be successful you must first learn to respect yourself, you deserve better. After all, your body is the only genuine temple the universe gave you. Now is the time to dig up all those deep rooted weeds which are slowly killing you. You must start communicating with your inner elephant, the Ganesha (the mover of all obstacles), once his course has been altered, you can sit on his back and have an easy ride into the future.

The next seven days after your first new moon fast is the most important time for shedding off old unwanted habits. Just like the female menstrual cycle, where the period sheds out unwanted material, your subconscious can do the same. For the next seven days you must stay focused on your new path. Your will power must be strong, as those bad habitual weeds are still rooted. The fast will have broken your routine, giving you space to go to work on your subconscious garden, you are once again in control, but you must keep focused for the next seven days until the first quarter moon appears. Positive thoughts towards your new goals must be reinforced at every opportunity, together with thoughts, visualisations and mantras, which will undermine and detach you from old unhealthy habits. Look in the mirror and be repulsed, look at others who are obese and be repulsed, get angry with yourself for letting it happen, whatever you can do to pull yourself away from those old habits for seven days you must do. Find new interests, new activities and visit new places, all in an effort to distract the mind from feeding the bad wolf and falling back into old habits. Instead of reaching for the coke, when thirsty, try one of many teas from all over the world. Instead of making a sandwich have a piece of fruit. Instead of sitting in front of the TV go for a walk. Make today the first day of the rest of your life.

"Seven days thou shalt eat unleavened bread, and in the seventh day shall be a feast to the Lord. Unleavened bread shall be eaten seven days; and there shall no leavened bread be seen with thee, neither shall there be leaven seen with thee in all thy quarters." - Exodus 13 : 6-7 (KJV)

"Do not leave the entrance to the tent of meeting for seven days, until the days of your ordination are completed, for your ordination will last seven days." - Leviticus 8 : 33 (NIV)

"After he is cleansed, he must wait seven days." - Ezekiel 44 : 26 (NIV)

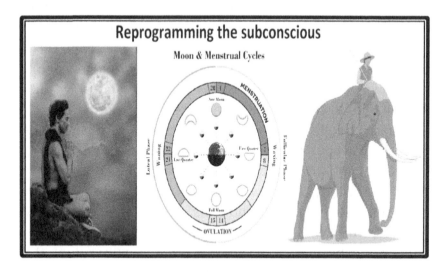

Reprogramming the subconscious

Moon & Menstrual Cycles

I am slim, happy, healthy

Eating disorders

There are many different eating disorders which disrupt an individuals eating patterns, some so severe they can lead to serious health issues. The most common disorders are:

- Anorexia Nervosa : A fear of gaining weight, with a perverted perception of self image. Although many sufferers are under weight, they still consider themselves to be fat or over weight.

- Bulimia Nervosa : This condition promotes binge eating followed by self induced vomiting, excessive exercise or the use of drugs to counteract the excessive bingeing and consumption of large amounts of calories.

- Binge eating : This is characterised by a loss of self control over normal eating habits. The individual will binge to excess periodically without implementing counter measures which Bulimia involves. Consequently, this disorder can pile on the weight fast.

The underlying causes behind eating disorders are many, a combination of psychological, environmental and biological factors, all playing a role in undermining a person's happy and contented disposition, ultimately going some way towards precipitating unhealthy eating habits.

The psychological factors which promote eating disorders usually come in the form of low self esteem and/or a negative perception of body image. This can be the result of trauma or abuse suffered during their formative years. Social pressures also contribute towards an expectation to look a certain way. These factors can become pronounced when a biological imbalance is added to the mix, expressing the individual's personality type through a particular eating disorder.

Damaged people subconsciously try to protect themselves from what they see as a bad unsafe world by putting on weight due to aspects of subconscious programming. Once this occurs, new behavioral patterns will start to germinate within the subconscious, leading to an unhealthy habit which can ruin a person's life. This is why the new moon fasting procedure is so important, as a way of initiating the break from bad habits for both the mind and body. It is vitally important with eating disorders that the underlining cause, fueling the behavior is dealt with. Sometimes it is necessary to remove yourself from whatever environmental factors are stimulating those psychological beliefs underpinning the disorder. A fresh start with a whole new way of thinking may be needed.

The power of collective meditation (the Maharishi effect).

To create the right environment for prayer to be effective it must always begin by centering oneself through the act of meditation.

Many people go to church, or their chosen place of worship, to rattle off vain repetitions of prayers which they have memorised from childhood, prayers which they automatically recite unconsciously. They do this without involving any form of meditation, rendering their prayers ineffective. The whole purpose of affirmative prayer is to change our conscious perspective from within. With intent we align both the sub and focal consciousness towards a given frequency and desired goal.

When someone tries to give up smoking after 20 years, they have great difficulty persuading their subconscious, the habitual mind, to quit. Although the focal conscious mind has decided to quit, the subconscious has been offered 20 years of affirming behaviour, telling it that it loves to smoke. By centering oneself in meditation, reprogramming the subconscious becomes much easier. Prayer and positive intentions towards the new "non-smoker" can be introduced planting new seeds and a new belief system, which in turn creates a new reality. When a group of people come together and focus their intention through group meditation some impressive results can be obtained. This is known as the Maharishi Effect.

During the summer of 1993, a controlled study was carried out in Washington DC, designed to see if a large group of 4,000 transcendental meditators could influence the city's crime rate. The meditators would, over a period of 8 weeks, use their calming influence over the cities inhabitants. Remarkably after the results were compiled, they discovered that the crime rate had indeed fallen by a staggering 23%.[7]

"The more self-critical and judgemental you are, the more your subconscious will work to convince you of your worthlessness. But if you make a habit of surrounding yourself with positive reminders and vibes, then the same thoughts will direct your actions towards goal orienting behaviour." - Rakhi Chakraborty[8]

Happy and healthy

It is well known that people with a natural happy disposition tend to live healthier lives than their miserable counterparts. Happiness, optimism and joviality are characteristics associated with Jupiter (Jove), whereas pessimism, loss, frustration and depression are character traits of Saturn (Satan).

"There is no path to happiness: happiness is the path." - Buddha

"Want to feel better and improve your health? Start by focusing on the things that bring you happiness. Scientific evidence suggests that positive emotions can help make life longer and healthier." - Harvard Medical School[9]

One step towards happiness is to accept ourselves in the present, be comfortable in our biological shells, and be at peace and harmony with body, soul and spirit. By accepting the self optimistically in the now we can avoid a life of Saturnian self accusation and denial, enabling all necessary emotional needs to be satisfied from within one's own mind. Those people who are unhappy in the now have placed false conditions upon their present well being, usually finding solace in some form of material acquisition. The now is not progress driven, it is therefore non-materialistic with no conditions or expectations placed on happiness. Many unhappy people have developed a belief system which requires conditions to be fulfilled in order for them to be happy, conditions such as:

- I will be happy at X point in the future.
- I will be happy when I have finished X.
- I will be happy when I have acquired X.
- I will be happy when I have accumulated X amount of money.

These are all saturnine constraints socially engineered as tools of division to keep society fragmented. How we see ourselves from within is far more important than what we do. If a person can be happy in all the 'NOWS' which make up their human experience, they will have a more pleasurable journey along the way, with the world smiling back at them. By being happy in the now, we can focus better, feel better, relate with others better and be more productive. It is all up to the individual's attitude.

"You must live in the present, launch yourself on every wave, find your eternity in each moment." - Henry David Thoreau

"I, not events, have the power to make me happy or unhappy today. I can choose which it shall be. Yesterday is dead, tomorrow hasn't arrived yet. I have just one day, today, and I'm going to be happy in it." - Groucho Marx

"We're so busy watching out for what's just ahead of us that we don't take time to enjoy where we are." - Bill Watterson

"Life is a preparation for the future; and the best preparation for the future is to live as if there were none." - Albert Einstein

"The here and now is all we have, and if we play it right it's all we'll need." - Ann Richards

"Are you responding to the NOW or reacting to your past?" - Ramana Pemmaraju

"Unease, anxiety, tension, stress, worry — all forms of fear — are caused by too much future, and not enough presence. Guilt, regret, resentment, grievances, sadness, bitterness, and all forms of non-forgiveness are caused by too much past, and not enough presence." - Eckhart Tolle

"Remember then: there is only one time that is important-- Now! It is the most important time because it is the only time when we have any power" - Leo Tolstoy

"The ability to be in the present moment is a major component of mental wellness." - Abraham Maslow

The average life of a person in the west is one of living within the constraints of Cronus (time), battling against the clock, forsaking all their "NOWS" for a romantic projection of themselves in the future, where they will be happy when they have "X", or shaken off the shackles of wage slavery by paying off all their debts; competing against one another within a narrow band of possibilities. Most of the human race are trapped in an endless cycle of compliance by their limited imaginations and programmed beliefs, along with their Darwinian desire to be better than their counterparts. They unwittingly compete to construct their own cells of suppression, eagerly imposing that suppression on their brothers and sisters. Most of them cannot fully accept or appreciate themselves in the "NOW" because they are worried about what others think of them, conditioned and domesticated towards the need to fit in, an expectation or preconceived idea as to what the norms are within their social surroundings and straight jackets of political correctness. To relieve the tension that builds up in their daily routine, many of them turn to alcohol, a false spirit offered by Saturnian corporations to administer a brief euphoria and detachment from their controlled lives. Pornography is also freely available and widely distributed over the internet, in an attempt to suppress and control their natural kundalini along with its healing potential.

We are a society of fragile expressions of universal consciousness divided, either stressed out, drugged up, pissed off, pissed up, spaced out, fearful of the future or stuck in the past. Occasionally you will meet a person who will stand out, a contented spirit living in the now, happy in the present with a balanced conscious connection to body, soul and spirit, shining like a beacon in a room full of fading candles all blowing in the opposite direction.

"The truth is there is an amazing infinite knowledge within us called the subconscious mind put there by the Creator of the universe. When we understand the laws of the universe

and co-exist in harmony with these undeniable truths, we can tap into this power and heal ourselves." - Dr Jill Carnahan MD[10]

Notes for chapter 5

(1) Dorothy Foltz-Gray, How depression hurts your health, 2016,
http://www.lifescript.com/health/centers/depression/articles/10_ways_depression_hurts_your_health.aspx

(2) Anthony Zappia, What's your frequency?
https://www.wellbeing.com.au/body/health/whats-your-frequency.html

(3) Your Rife Machine History Educational Website.
http://www.rifevideos.com/index.html

(4) Martin Enserink, Can the placebo be the cure?, Science, sciencemag.org, 1999.
http://science.sciencemag.org/content/284/5412/238

(5) Professor Damien Finniss, medical doctor and Associate Professor at the University of Sydney's Pain Management and Research Institute. Interviewed by Paul Biegler, 'Mind-body' healing: Success of placebo trials challenges medical thinking, Healthcare, Sunday Morning Herald.
https://www.smh.com.au/healthcare/mindbody-healing-success-of-placebo-trials-challenges-medical-thinking-20170605-gwkk2c.html

(6) A controlled trial of arthroscopic surgery for osteoarthritis of the knee, The New England journal of medicine, July 11 2002

(7) John S. Hagelin, Maxwell V. Rainforth, David W. Orme-Johnson, Kenneth L. Cavanaugh, Charles N. Alexander, Susan F. Shatkin, John L. Davies, Anne O. Hughes, and Emanuel Ross, Effects of Group Practice of the Transcendental Meditation Program on Preventing Violent Crime in

Washington, DC: Results of the National Demonstration Project, June-July 1993, Institute of science technology and public policy. http://istpp.org/crime_prevention/

(8) Rakhi Chakraborty, How you can change your life by thinking. 2015, Yourstory. https://yourstory.com/2015/04/power-of-thoughts/

(9) The happiness health connection, Harvard Health Publishing, Harvard Medical School. https://www.health.harvard.edu/healthbeat/the-happiness-health-connection

(10) Dr Jill Carnahan MD, The power of the subconscious mind to heal you, 2016. https://www.jillcarnahan.com/2016/08/21/power-subconscious-mind-heal/

Chapter 6, metaphysical workout.

Those who understand astrology can appreciate the different characteristics associated with each sun-sign. Consequently, some exercise activities are more suitable to certain sun-signs than others . Each sign is assigned one of the four elements (fire, earth, air, water), together with the cardinal, fixed and mutable qualities of those signs. Aries for example, is a cardinal fire sign, ruled by the planet Mars. So anyone with this sun-sign (focal consciousness/soul) should be particularly suited to physically proactive and dynamic exercises, in a specific direction, which burn off calories, like cycling.

Cardinal : Starting something new or change of direction.

Fixed : The continuation of a process.

Mutable : A change or the ending of one process for the next.

Fire	Air
Fire : Passionate, Dynamic, Temperamental	Air : Action, Ideas, Motion
C : Spark	C : Breath of fresh air
F : Burning	F : Breeze
M : Ashes or Smolder	M : Winds of change

Earth	Water
Earth : Grounded, Stable, Practical	Water : Emotional, Sensitive, Intuitive
C : Ploughing the field	C : Rain
F : Solid foundations	F : Sea, lake or pond
M : Earthquake	M : Tides, shoreline, tsunami

Aries

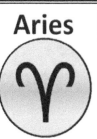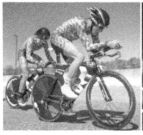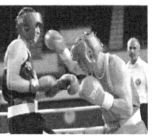

Cardinal Fire = Spark
Ruled by Mars (God of war), proactive energy in a direction.

Recommended activity : Cycling, Boxing .

Taurus

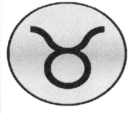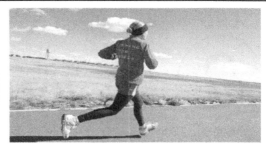

Fixed Earth = Solid foundations, slow and steady.
Ruled by Venus (love and liking).

Recommended activity : Running .

Gemini

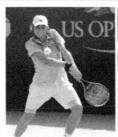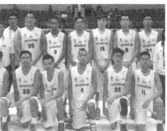

Mutable Air = Winds of change
Ruled by Mercury (communication), fast thinking.

Recommended activity : Tennis, Team sports.

Cancer

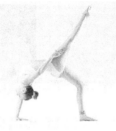
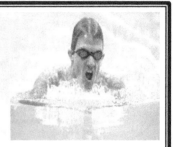

Cardinal Water = Rain
Ruled by the Moon (Emotion, sensitivity).

Recommended activity : Yoga, Swimming, Home workout.

Leo

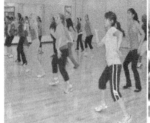
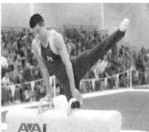

Fixed Fire = Burning
Ruled by the Sun (will, Soul, focal consciousness).

Recommended activity : Dance cardio, competitive workouts, gymnastics.

Virgo

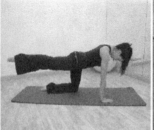
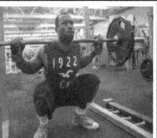

Mutable Earth = Earthquake
Ruled by Mercury (communication).

Recommended activity : Pilates, weight training, hard short burst exercises.

Libra

 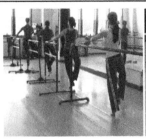 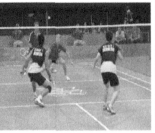

Cardinal Air = Breath of fresh air
Ruled by Venus (love and liking).

Recommended activity : Balancing exercises (barre),
companion exercises, badminton.

Sagittarius

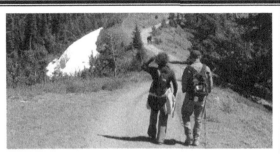

Mutable Fire = Ashes
Ruled by Jupiter (optimism, abundance).
Recommended activity : Hiking, outdoor and on the move.

Scorpio

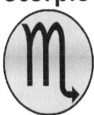 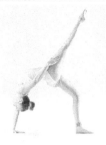 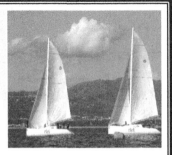

Fixed Water = Sea, lake, pond
Ruled by Mars (proactive energy).

Recommended activity : Yoga, Sailing and water-sports.

Capricorn

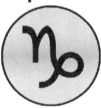 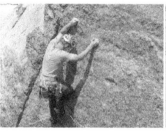 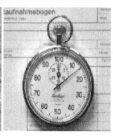

Cardinal Earth = Ploughing the field
Ruled by Saturn (order and control).

Recommended activity : Rock climbing, Endurance,
discipline, time restraints.

Aquarius

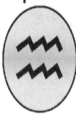 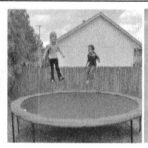 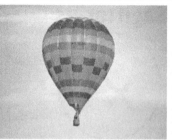

Fixed Air : Breeze
Ruled by Saturn (order & control) Uranus (out of the blue, new technology)
Recommended activity : Trampolining, parachuting, hang-gliding, hot air balloon.

Pisces

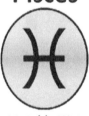 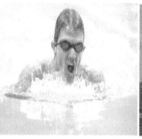 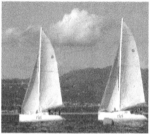

Mutable Water : Tides
Ruled by Jupiter (optimism, abundance).
Recommended activity : Swimming, water-sports.

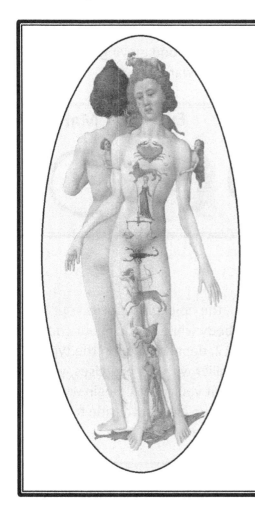

Aries - Head

Taurus - Throat
Gemini - Arms
Cancer - Chest
Leo - Heart
Virgo - Gut
Libra - Kidneys
Scorpio - Genitals

Sagittarius - Hips

Capricorn - Knees

Aquarius - Shins

Pisces - Feet

As the human body is reflected within all twelve signs of the zodiac, it makes sense, when creating a full body workout, to take this into consideration. When the Sun comes up on the horizon (horus rising) its soul consciousness/rays energise our own conscious perspective, by pulling us back into focal awareness, from the world of the subconscious/spirit realm. We awaken and open our eyes, to once again view and interact with this physical reality. Starting in Aries we begin a new zodiac cycle going through all the signs, ending in Pisces.

Consequently, during the hours of 6am to 8am, the planet Mars is dominant, ruling the sign of Aries. Mars is the planet of proactive energy, so to be in tune with nature some form of exercise is recommended to get the blood moving and to fully pull us into a higher sense of focal awareness.

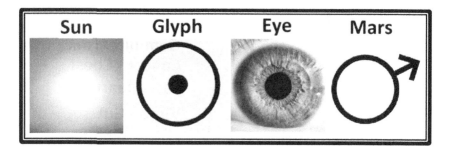

| Sun | Glyph | Eye | Mars |

Aries, head exercises

Starting at the top of the head, the object is to focus your full attention on each area of the body while reciting your chosen mantra. Do this in sets of 4 or 12, depending upon the type of exercise. Once you become familiar with the exercises, you can customise the workout to suit your needs. Begin with simple eye exercises, move them up and down, side to side, and in circles, one way and then the other.

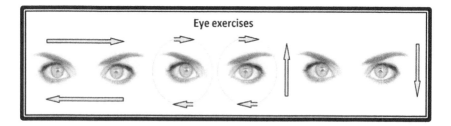

Eye exercises

Nose

The stimulating breath technique is used to boost alertness by increasing the air flow into the lungs. Visualise your lungs as bellows, while breathing in and out rapidly in short bursts.

Repeat 1 cycle of 12, 4 times. Be careful the increased oxygen does not make you too light headed. After performing this you should feel more alert and awake.

Ears

With your mouth closed make a fog horn sound in the throat which vibrates throughout the head, especially in the ears. Find the correct pitch which will almost tickle the inner ear. Repeat this 12 times visualising the "OM" sound.

Taurus, neck exercises

The neck exercises are similar to those for the eye. Begin by standing firmly on the ground, with your legs slightly apart. Look left and right while chanting your mantra. Repeat this by looking up and down, then side to side, taking care you don't over stretch and cause discomfort.

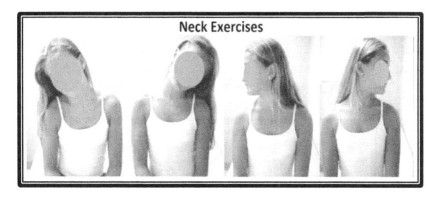
Neck Exercises

Gemini, arm exercises

There are many arm exercises available, here are just a few simple ones which can easily be done at home. Follow on from the neck exercises, with the feet already in the correct position, arm circles can be performed. Stretch your arms out, both sides, and begin to move them in large circles, one way and then the other. This can be done 12 times while reciting positive mantra. Push-ups are another favourite with variations in the positioning of the hands, either close together or far apart, for extra difficulty. If you find this too difficult, wall or bed push-ups on an incline are an easier alternative.

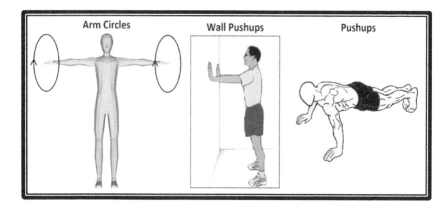

Cancer, chest exercises

Along with push-ups, hand clasps are an easy option when exercising the chest. Simply clasp your hands together, out in front of you, while tensing the chest muscles for a period of time. This will exercise the chest without straining.

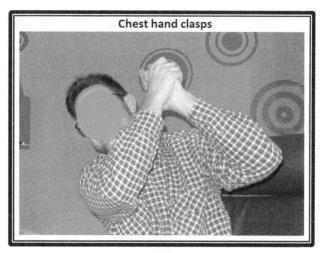

Leo, heart and high abs

One of the main contributors to heart disease is excessive weight and lack of physical exercise. So it is important that this is addressed as soon as possible in order to begin the process of becoming the best version of yourself. A couple of simple exercises will focus on the higher abs below the chest. The first is the knee crunch, where the individual lays on their back with the legs bent and knees up. Either with arms crossed over the chest or out stretched above the head, bring your arms and top part of the body up and forward towards the knees. Repeat this 12 times as slow as physically possible, concentrating on the upper abs. The other exercise in this section concentrates on the back, it is known as the superman for obvious reasons. Simply lay on the floor and stretch your arms and legs out and up, as though your flying like superman, tensing all the muscles to the back of the body. Hold this position for 4 counts of your chosen mantra.

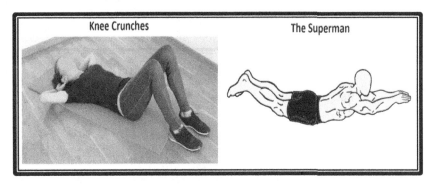

Knee Crunches   The Superman

Virgo, lower abs

Two exercises are recommended for this part of the body, leg raises and the elbow plank. For leg raises simply lay on your back and gently raise your legs up off the ground for an extended period of time. The second exercise is to turn yourself over laying on the floor supported by your forearms and toes. It is referred to as the elbow plank because as you flex your abs your body becomes rigid like a plank.

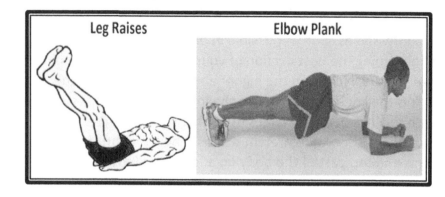

Libra, lower back

For the lower back a variation to the superman can be performed, called the alternate superman. Once in the superman position lift one arm along with the opposite leg, repeat this numerous times with both arms and legs reciting mantra.

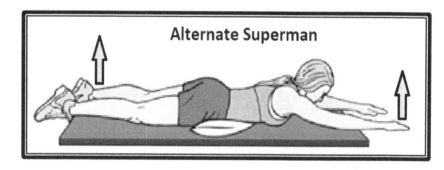

Scorpio, groin and buttocks

To strengthen the groin area the exercise known as the adductor squeeze can be performed. Simply lay on the floor with a ball or cushion between your knees and gently squeeze flexing the groin muscles. Repeat 12 times holding for the time it takes to recite your mantra. For the buttocks, reverse leg raises are simple but effective. Start off in either the elbow plank position or with both knees on the ground as an easier option, lift one leg at a time, by stretching it up and back. Repeat this 12 times with both legs until your happy you have worked enough on that area. This will exercise and flex your buttocks without putting strain on other areas of the body.

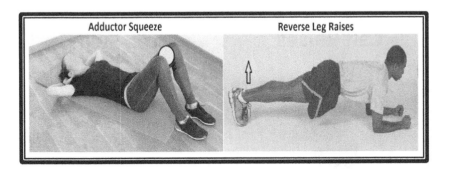

Adductor Squeeze | Reverse Leg Raises

Sagittarius, Hips and thighs

Simply walking on the spot, lifting each leg relatively high is a perfect exercise for the home environment. Occasionally throwing in a hip circle. This is where the knee goes up and out, creating a circle in the air, exercising the hip joint. Also do this in reverse where the knee goes out sideways first then back in-front, producing a reverse circle.

Capricorn, Knee caps and skeletal system

Loosen up by moving all your joints, wiggle your fingers and toes, along with stretching your arms to almost touching the ceiling. Bend your knees and shake yourself down before moving on to the next exercise.

Aquarius, calves, shins and ankles

Calf raises. While standing on your feet slowly lift yourself up onto your toes, flexing the calf muscles. Hold this position while reciting your mantra, then release back down to the start position, repeating this process 12 times. To exercise the ankles simply stand on one foot and swing the other leg in a random pendulum fashion, keeping your balance as you go. This puts emphasis on the ankle, strengthening it in the process.

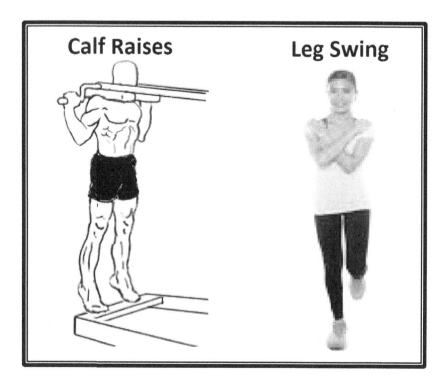

Calf Raises   **Leg Swing**

Pisces, feet

To complete the zodiac workout lay on the floor and focus on your feet. Move the feet and the toes around freely while continuing to recite your chosen mantra. This can be done In sets of 12 seconds.

You have now completed a full metaphysical body workout, now is an ideal time to jump in the shower to enjoy the sensation of water flowing over your body. This should stimulate the subconscious with a positive sensation, as a reward for the effort just undertaken. Stand, relax and meditate while the water is dropping all around you. Try to keep focused on the moment and the sensations you are experiencing along with your breath and the mantra you are still reciting. This will all work in your favour towards new positive intentions and new behavioral patterns, which will transform your old unhealthy habits into new horizons. Initially, you must have the strength of character and will power to take back the reins of control over your life, building on your own unique perspective of reality. Only you see the world from your unique perspective, and it is only you who can rise above social pressures to become the best version of yourself. Be that independent candle which shines on its own merits, brighter and taller than all those who have lost control.

Chapter 7, relocation and cosmic influence.

Be careful who you mix with, as their influence within your particular proximity will ultimately play a part in your overall behaviour. Your perception of physical reality is formulated within the mind as parameters of focal consciousness. Our five senses pick up and feed us only a limited view from those energy vibrations which surround us. With more senses a greater level of awareness can be experienced, unfortunately most of the frequency vibrations are beyond our biological ability to perceive, making us almost blind in a universe of infinite energetic potential and possibility. A person's birth chart is an important guide to their personality type and the potential of conscious interaction within this universal construct. Although the zodiac is commonly used to view planetary influences within time, it can also be used as a guide of planetary influences over proximity, especially concerning the Earth. The position of the planets within the birth chart can be transposed over the geography of the Earth, placing planetary energetic emphasis on specific areas. For example if you live in a city under the influence of Jupiter, its overall characteristics are more likely to play a significant role in your day to day living, with the potential to expand your waist line. This type of astrology is known as astrocartography.

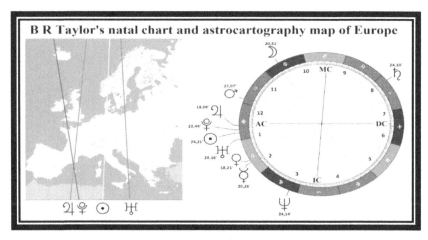

B R Taylor's natal chart and astrocartography map of Europe

The astrocartographic map is produced using the birth place as the benchmark for its calculations. The previous picture is an example of how an astrocartographic map is constructed from the information taken from an individual's natal chart. We see Jupiter's path of influence, the first planet below the ascendant (AC), influencing specific areas with its unique characteristics of abundance, expansion, good fortune and optimism. Here the individual has the potential to pile the weight on, consequently, they must be careful not to fall into bad eating habits. From this data one can identify those areas on the planet which offer natural karmic influences in all aspects of life, for example if a person is looking for love, it would make sense to move to those areas which fall under the influence of Venus, the planet of love and liking. If a person wishes to be popular, creative and full of vitality, using this system, it would be advantageous for them to move to an area heavily influenced by the Sun.

A line's influence is stronger the closer one is to it, but this doesn't mean the other planets cease to have any effect. It is generally accepted that a line's energy will have an influence of up to 200km away. There is a symphony of energies all mixing together with transiting planets and aspects all playing a role. Although astrocartography, in its modern form, is in its infancy, it can still offer us some interesting insights.

Oliver Hardy's astrocartographic map

Oliver Hardy was a comedy actor during the early years of Hollywood. He paired up with Stan Laurel to form one of Americas most famous double acts known as Laurel and Hardy. They began in the days of silent movies, with their last performance being in 1955. Oliver Hardy died in August 1957 from complications resulting from a stroke.

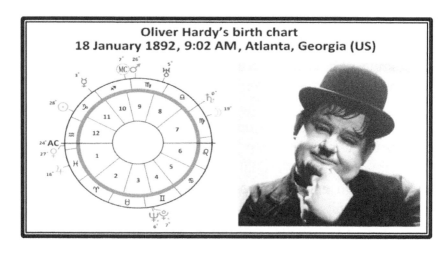

Oliver Hardy's birth chart
18 January 1892, 9:02 AM, Atlanta, Georgia (US)

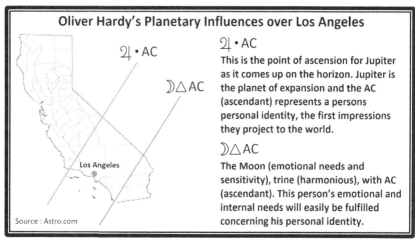

Oliver Hardy's Planetary Influences over Los Angeles

♃ • AC

♄ • AC

☽ △ AC

Los Angeles

Source : Astro.com

♃ • AC

This is the point of ascension for Jupiter as it comes up on the horizon. Jupiter is the planet of expansion and the AC (ascendant) represents a persons personal identity, the first impressions they project to the world.

☽ △ AC

The Moon (emotional needs and sensitivity), trine (harmonious), with AC (ascendant). This person's emotional and internal needs will easily be fulfilled concerning his personal identity.

Oliver Hardy lived in Los Angeles from the early 1920s.[1] His natal chart's planetary influence over this part of the world gives rise to the potential for weight gain, being subject to both the energy from the Moon and Jupiter.

Aretha Franklin's astrocartographic map

Aretha Franklin was an American singer who became known as "The Queen of Soul" after a string of hits during the 1960s. Aretha was born in Memphis Tennessee in March 1942, after which her family moved to Detroit when she was 5 years old.

After she had established herself in the music business she returned to Detroit in the early 1980s, which became her home till she died of pancreatic cancer in August 2018.

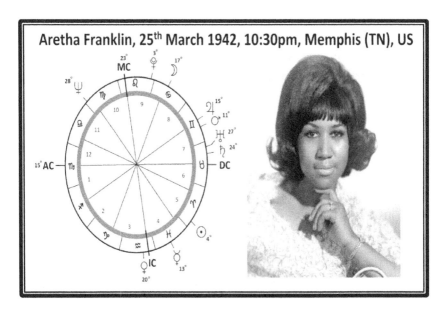

Aretha Franklin, 25th March 1942, 10:30pm, Memphis (TN), US

Aretha Franklin spent most of her life being overweight, at 34 she lost 40 lbs on an intensive crash diet, only to put it all back on over the next few years. Excess weight is a major contributing factor towards pancreatic cancer.[2]

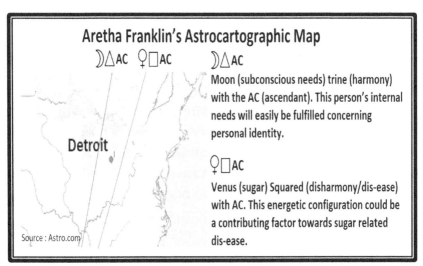

Aretha Franklin's Astrocartographic Map

☽△AC ♀□AC

Detroit

Source : Astro.com

☽△AC

Moon (subconscious needs) trine (harmony) with the AC (ascendant). This person's internal needs will easily be fulfilled concerning personal identity.

♀□AC

Venus (sugar) Squared (disharmony/dis-ease) with AC. This energetic configuration could be a contributing factor towards sugar related dis-ease.

The interesting part of Aretha Franklin's astrocartographic map is the Venus squared AC, which could have had a contributing influence towards her problem with diabetes.

"In 2014, Ms. Franklin disclosed to a local news station that she had diabetes, but did not specify in the interview if she were diagnosed with type 1 diabetes or type 2 diabetes." - GluCraig[3]

The energetic influence which the planets have over our lives effects us in a number of ways:

- Our natal chart (karmic disposition).
- Planetary transits (day to day movement of the planets).
- Our proximity on this Earth.

Some people may find that in order to avoid specific weight gaining macrocosmic stimuli, they would benefit from a relocation or an overall change in environment. This also makes it easier to break old habits and bring forward new ones.

Gemstones

In some ancient religious and philosophical practices, such as Hinduism and Buddhism, it is believed that life on Earth is influenced by nine different mechanisms, known as "Navaratna" (the nine influences). This turns out to be the seven ancient planets together with the north and south nodes of the Moon. Each influence was given a specific gemstone, which supposedly replicated the unique characteristics and qualities of those nine planets. The gemstones chosen can be seen on pages 152 & 153, with Hessonite and Cats eye, as additions, representing the north and south nodes of the Moon respectively.

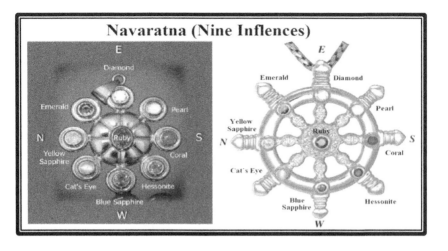

Navaratna (Nine Inflences)

Because the gemstones were thought to be fixed reflections of planetary energies, as time went by, people would wear various stones believing they would enhance certain aspects of their lives. Each positive experience would reinforce the belief in the power of the gemstone, Whether due to genuine metaphysical qualities or not, if the individual believed in its power it could certainly contribute to the placebo effect.

Rings & fingers

Once the significance of each stone is understood, along with the unique energetic characteristics associated with them, one can utilise these energies, targeting specific areas of one's life. The fingers are believed to act as antennae, receivers to outside frequencies and universal energy. Each finger has its own karmic disposition according to one's own planetary natal configuration. To amplify, offset or stimulate areas of concern, one can place specific gemstones on various fingers in order to create the correct energetic balance required for particular goals, wants and needs. Just as the subconscious is influenced by our thoughts and feelings, our receptivity to planetary transits can be enhanced using a selection of gemstones in the right places. This concept is fully explained in my book 'Metaphysics of the Gods'.

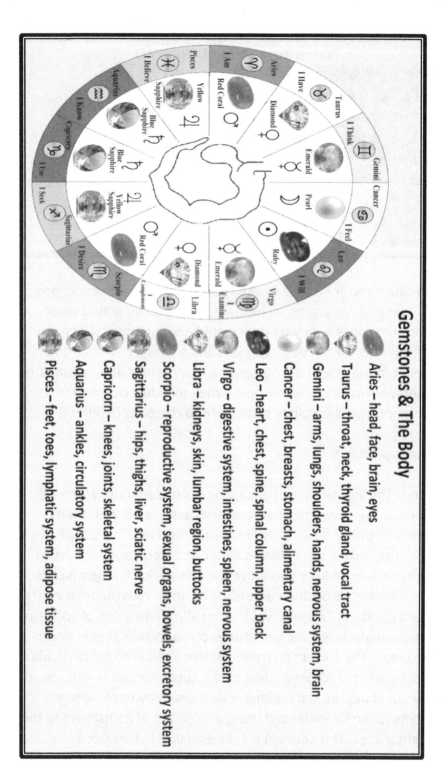

Gemstones & The Body

Aries – head, face, brain, eyes

Taurus – throat, neck, thyroid gland, vocal tract

Gemini – arms, lungs, shoulders, hands, nervous system, brain

Cancer – chest, breasts, stomach, alimentary canal

Leo – heart, chest, spine, spinal column, upper back

Virgo – digestive system, intestines, spleen, nervous system

Libra – kidneys, skin, lumbar region, buttocks

Scorpio – reproductive system, sexual organs, bowels, excretory system

Sagittarius – hips, thighs, liver, sciatic nerve

Capricorn – knees, joints, skeletal system

Aquarius – ankles, circulatory system

Pisces – feet, toes, lymphatic system, adipose tissue

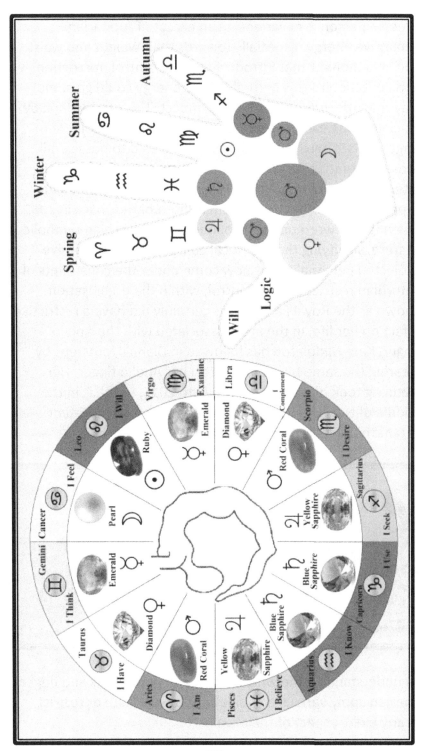

When a person is experiencing an excess of Jupitarian expansive energy, especially towards their weight and waist line, it is thought that introducing more control, restriction and limitation to this natural cosmic energy could go some way towards reducing its overall impact. This can be done by placing a blue sapphire on either the Jupiter or Apollo(Sun) finger. This is because a blue sapphire is said to possess all those energetic characteristics associated with Saturn. It is interesting to point out that Princess Diana received a blue sapphire engagement ring, from Prince Charles, back in 1981. The ring was worn on her Apollo finger, a Saturnian symbolic gesture, signifying that her focal conscious and expressive projected personality has now come under the constraints of Saturnian restriction and control, within the organisation known as the Royal Family. This certainly did have a restrictive effect on her life, in the areas associated with the Apollo finger. Kate Middleton has followed in Diana's footsteps by wearing the same blue sapphire on her Apollo finger. Her wedding took place on April the 29th 2011, which is in the middle of the "Grand Climax", one of the most important Satanic holidays of the year.[4]

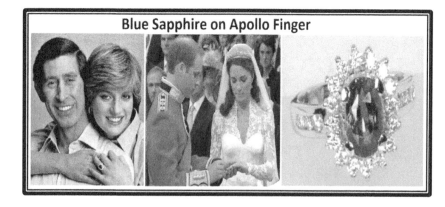

Blue Sapphire on Apollo Finger

By understanding the whole concept of gemstones and fingers one can apply various combinations to stimulate or restrict nearly every aspect of their lives.

Notes for chapter 7

(1) Oliver Hardy's home, Los Angeles. History's Homes.
http://www.historyshomes.com/detail.cfm?id=425

(2) Gabe Mirkin, Aretha Franklin struggled with weight gain during her brilliant career, 2018. Village News.
https://www.villages-news.com/aretha-franklin-struggled-with-weight-gain-during-her-brilliant-career/

(3) Craig Idlebrook / GluCraig, Aretha Franklin, who had diabetes, passes away. Aug 2018, Glu.
https://myglu.org/articles/aretha-franklin-who-had-diabetes-passes-away

(4) List of satanic holidays, the open scroll,
http://www.theopenscroll.com/hosting/SatanicCalendar.htm

Conclusion

When considering that astrology is the oldest living language known to man, its synchronised wisdom is so profound that it truly is the benchmark expressing our relationship with nature. Consequently, if humanity is to restore its place and direction here on Earth, by living in harmony with nature's rhythms and cycles, it must go back to some of the old ways, appreciating the cosmos and the solar system as a whole. The early Gnostic Christians understood the importance of astrology. The Bible makes a clear reference to the constellation Pleiades having an influence on us. It also mentions the Mazzaroth in the book of Job, Mazzaroth is an old Biblical Hebrew term which refers to the zodiac.

"Canst thou bind the sweet influences of Pleiades, or loose the bands of Orion? Canst thou bring forth Mazzaroth in his season? Or canst thou guide Arcturus with his sons. Knowest thou the ordinances of heaven? Canst thou set the dominion thereof in the earth?" - Job 38: 31-33 (KJV)

The word 'Mazzaroth' is only used once in the Bible, it is thought to be referring to the zodiac. However in the KJV version it is quite specific as to the "sweet influences of the Pleiades", it is therefore clear that the writers of the Bible at that time understood that the constellations of the zodiac had an influence on humanity.

"The word's precise meaning is uncertain but its context is that of astronomical constellations, and it is often interpreted as a term for the zodiac or the constellations thereof" - Mazzaroth, Wikipedia[1]

According to the New International Bible this is what the Lord said:

"Stand at the crossroads and look; ask for the ancient paths, ask where the good way is, and walk in it, and you will find rest for your souls. But you said, 'We will not walk in it.'" - Jeremiah 6 : 16 (NIV)

The crossroads refer to the four cardinal points of the zodiac. The ancient path or "the way" is what the early Gnostic Christians would call themselves, followers of "the way". And those who rejected the way were in danger of bringing dis-harmony and dis-ease upon their souls.

"Meanwhile, Saul was still breathing out murderous threats against the Lord's disciples. He went to the high priest and asked him for letters to the synagogues in Damascus, so that if he found any there who belonged to The Way, whether men or women, he might take them as prisoners to Jerusalem." - Acts 9 : 1-2 (NIV)

How we perceive and interact with the world around us is a reflection of our focal and subconscious beliefs, wants and needs. And those mechanisms which programmed our initial beliefs are ultimately behind humanity's future direction. If you fail to understand this and take back control over your own subconscious programming those mechanisms will do it for you. Although positive intent has the potential to initiate new beliefs which can overturn bad habits, in order to fully embrace the universal law of attraction one needs to be proactive by launching oneself wholeheartedly towards one's new direction. The relationship between the universe and your part in it is a co-creation, and for the law of attr-action to work, you must get up, out and about, fulfilling the action part of the co-creation. They say the universe will give you what you need but not necessarily what you want, so when you spring into action with a new positive belief, in yourself and the future, you will find people, places and events will help you along the way as the universe conspires behind the scenes to make your new objectives come true.

As we move further into this new Age of Aquarius, Saturn, the ruler in traditional astrology, will promote more control, restriction and order in nearly every aspect of our lives. While on the other hand Uranus, a planet synonymous with opposing characteristics to Saturn will share ruler-ship for the first 1000 years.

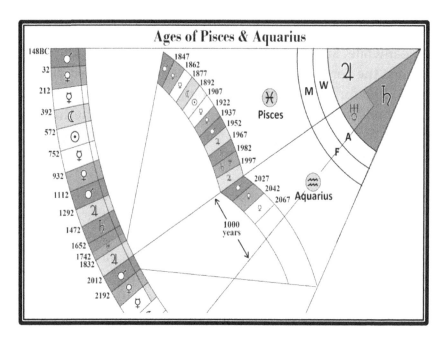

The freedoms of Uranus are contrary to the restrictive controls associated with Saturn. This will no doubt offer the human experience a great deal of contrasting options, depending upon which side you are on, or which spectrum of energies you align yourself with. Will you become part of the control system, embracing and underpinning all its artificial constructs, or will you break free, uniting with nature, to live a more fulfilled and harmonious life, enjoying nature's bounty, good health and an optimistic vision for the future?

With Saturn, the cross of materialism over the crescent of spirituality, dominating the Age as its new ruling planet, materialism will take over from spirituality underpinning our new social foundations. Pulling humanity away from nature will become a priority to the Saturnian control system, which will lead most of the world's population towards transhumanism with artificial and materialistic goals.

Decimalisation has replaced the old numerical systems which were based on 12, the number of universal harmony. Decimalisation is based around 10, it is the 'X' shaped cross in Roman numerals, which in astrology represents a Grand Cross, the most harsh and inharmonious aspect an astrological chart can manifest. The Grand Cross depicts four planets squaring and opposing one another. Square aspects possess Mars like characteristics while oppositions are Saturnian in nature. The 10th house of the zodiac is Capricorn, the house of career, ruled by Saturn, its motto is "I use". The word sinister is Latin for left handed, and the left hand is also ruled by Saturn and the Moon (Sin).

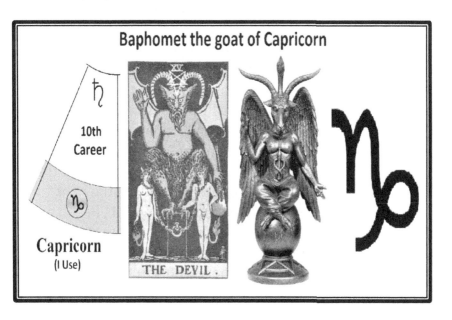

Baphomet the goat of Capricorn

10th Career

Capricorn
(I Use)

THE DEVIL.

Decem is Latin for ten	Words beginning with 'Dec'

X

Decay, Deceit, Decline, Deceive, Deceased, Decouple, Decrease, Decimate, Decadence, Decolonise, Deconstruct, Decompose.

To recap and consolidate. The metaphysical diet, in short, is not only a diet of what and when you eat, but more of a philosophical way of life, bringing you back from the brink of ill health and obesity towards a lighter more optimistic way of living.

I suspect, many people who have got this far through the book have at one time or another had some issues with weight gain, even to a point where they feel they have lost control over their eating habits. However, I suspect, many still hold onto an optimistic glimmer of hope in turning the situation around. If this is to happen, it is important to focus on that positive optimism, which can stimulate the will into changing direction, from unhealthy eating habits into positive new ones. With a strong belief that 'thy will be done' all is possible hear on Earth, just as it is in heaven. All you need to do is follow these simple steps, as each step is one progression in the right direction and part of a new path towards wealth, health and happiness. It is also important to be aware of the Moon's phases and look forward to the next new moon, as a golden opportunity to connect once more with nature and your universally given divine heritage.

From all those who contributed to this books conception, we wish you the best of luck and success. Strive to be happy and strive to be the best version of yourself.

Basic rules of the metaphysical diet

- **Do not break your fast until Noon.**
- **Try to stick to only eating between 12-2pm. If you must graze in the evening eat low (GL) foods.**
- **Fast on a new moon day, and meditate concentrating on the house of the zodiac your new moon falls into and use a mantra reflecting the characteristics of that house and the changes you want to see in your life.**
- **When exercising use positive mantra and natural zodiacal numerical cycles (12 & 4).**

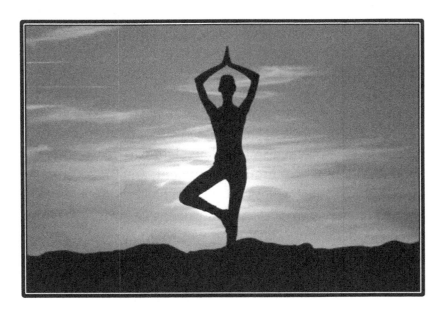

Notes for Conclusion

(1) Mazzaroth, Wikipedia,

Author's Bio

Brian Taylor was born in a small town in the suburbs of Nottingham, England during the late 1960s. After graduating with BSc (Hons) in construction management from Leeds Polytechnic in 1992, he spent most of his time working as an engineer. After many years fascinated by the bigger questions of life, he chose to take time away from western society, to pursue a journey of discovery. With an open mind and an optimistic belief in himself, he decided to see where destiny would take him.

During his many years travelling mostly throughout Southeast Asia, he discovered the answers to many of the questions which he had been carrying for years. At this time he wrote two books, the first one entitled *'Language of the Gods'*, was a comprehensive breakdown of how the controlling elite divide and rule humanity from a physical perspective, with an astrological overtone. His second book *'Metaphysics of the Gods'* looked into how universal energies are the building blocks for our perception of reality, within a feed-back loop of human consciousness. At this stage in his journey, he began to understand the mechanisms in play relating to how we influence our reality. A profound moment, and the most important and valuable lesson an individual can learn in a limited lifetime. From this core knowledge he revisited history to see if it made more sense. This was when he wrote *'Metaphysics of WW2'*.

As the years progressed Mr Taylor noticed an increase in obesity in western tourists visiting Southeast Asia. American and British tourists in particular, appeared to have developed some unhealthy eating habits in comparison to the Asians, who, on the whole, ate a relatively healthy and modest diet. This prompted Mr Taylor to investigate the subject from a metaphysical perspective, not only to benefit others, but also himself. This resulted in the book *'The Metaphysical Diet'*. To add to the series of books on metaphysics and suspecting that humanity was being steered in a direction which was not entirely righteous Mr Taylor next decided to investigate Kabbalah in relation to astrotheology and the globalisation project. This resulted in his book *'The Left Hand Path'*.

Finally, after more years of travelling and still evermore fascinated and puzzled by life's deeper questions, Mr Taylor focused on research regarding our connection to the spirit realm. This resulted in the book *'When The Spirit Takes Over'*.

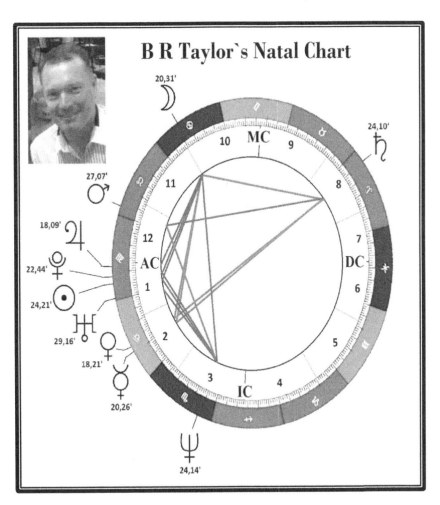

Other books by this author

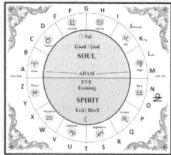

This book sets out to challenge the way we see the world, our adopted belief systems and coordinates within world history. It exposes how the potential of a united humanity has been suppressed by various forms of control over thousands of years, elites which have used division in both our physical and spiritual realms. The book is a journey of discovery into our true connection to the universe, and the relationship between the macrocosm and microcosm. The reader will come away with a fresh empowering view of how planetary cycles and energies along with human consciousness are the drivers behind geopolitical events and the ever changing fortunes of time.

"We are what we think. All that we
are arises with our thoughts.
With our thoughts, we make the
world." Buddha

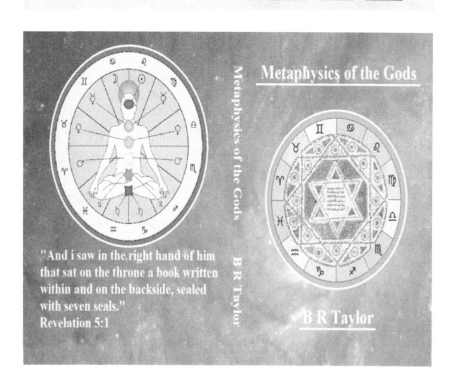

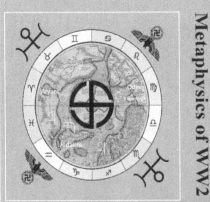

Metaphysics of WW2

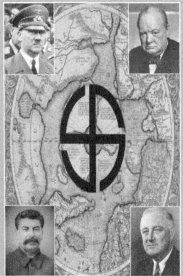

If you think you understand WW2, think again! Until you have looked into the metaphysical (beyond the physical) aspect of the subject, together with the astrological timing in which it took place, you really are only scratching the surface. Many war historians and scholars concern themselves with the people, places and events surrounding WW2, but neglect the bigger picture. This is the only book of its kind to give you the big picture.

Metaphysics of WW2

B R Taylor

B R Taylor

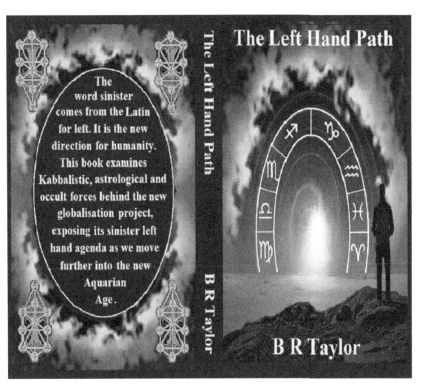

The Left Hand Path

The word sinister comes from the Latin for left. It is the new direction for humanity. This book examines Kabbalistic, astrological and occult forces behind the new globalisation project, exposing its sinister left hand agenda as we move further into the new Aquarian Age.

The Left Hand Path

B R Taylor

B R Taylor

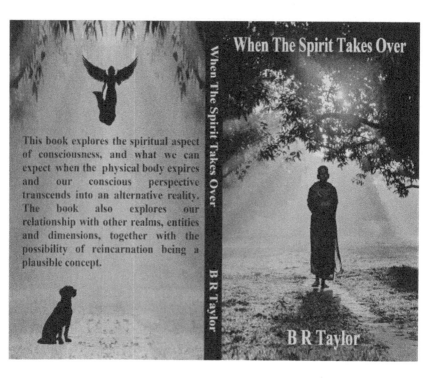

Websites by this author

www.BRTaylorMetaphysics.com

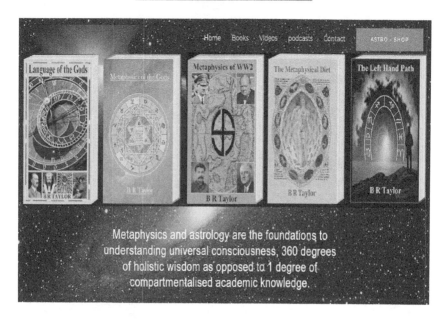

https://www.youtube.com/channel/UC6Ic7_8H0JGdrDhpQWuvfBQ

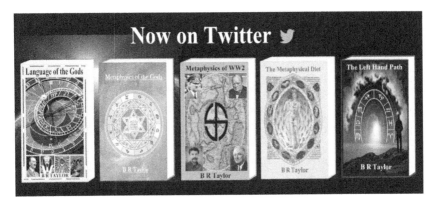

https://www.bitchute.com/channel/O60Mhc33iUmU/
https://brandnewtube.com/@BRTaylor
https://odysee.com/@BRTaylorMataphysics:b
https://twitter.com/BRTaylor14

.

Made in the USA
Las Vegas, NV
07 August 2023

75765049R00098